Minerals

Key to Vibrant Health and Life Force

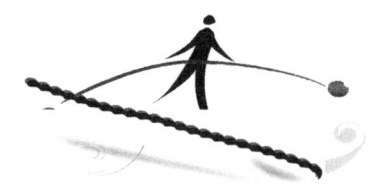

Jacob Swilling, Ph.D. BCHC

Consulting Research Scientist
Know Your Options™

Copyright © 2011, 2019 Jacob Swilling, Ph.D BCHC

KYO Publishing

No part of this book may be reproduced, transmitted, or reprinted in any form except for brief excerpts for the purpose of reviews, without the express written permission of the publisher at
kyopublishing@gmail.com

The information presented in this work is in no way intended as medical advice or as a substitute for medical counseling. The information herein should be used in conjunction with
the guidance and care of your
health professional, naturopath, or physician.

All rights reserved

Published by KYO Publishing
14252 Culver Drive #913
Irvine CA 92606
email: kyopublishing@gmail.com

First edition

ISBN# 978-0-9851369-2-5

Preface

We are generally familiar with certain minerals essential to health, such as iron, calcium, iodine, and zinc. But few of us are knowledgeable about all the other minerals which are essential for maintaining our bones, teeth, muscle, blood, and nerve cells. These inorganic elements and compounds are an essential part of a healthy diet. They occur naturally in nonliving things such as rocks and metal ores, as well as plants, which contain these elements from the soil. Minerals and vitamins work together to provide the nutrients we all need for healthy living.

Few individuals understand the nature and functions of minerals as well as Dr. Jacob Swilling. Having studied their effects on the body for the past twenty-five years, Dr. Swilling has crusaded to bring his comprehensive knowledge of the essential components of achieving good health naturally, without the use of pharmaceutical drugs on which so many people seem to depend.

This book is a companion to several others which Dr. Swilling has written, that reveal his vast knowledge of the life-giving qualities of nutrients, which have grown less abundant naturally, due to the depletion of our soils, and the addition of hundreds of questionable and often toxic chemicals which have been added to processed foods.

Dr. Swilling dedicates this and his other remarkable books to the continued health and well-being of all.

Contents

Chapter 1 - Introduction 1
   Neglected Area of Research 5
   Balancing Minerals 7

**Chapter 2 - A Review of Organic
and Homeopathic Minerals**.. 9

Chapter 3 - Overview of Minerals 21
   Trace Minerals 38
   Other Minerals 53

Chapter 4 - Cell Chemistry 61
   Drinking Water - Mineral Content of Water 69

Chapter 5 - The Synergistic Impact of Water.......... 69
   Balance and Osmosis 73
   Water Intoxication 75
   Impact of Dehydration on Cancer 76
   Water Movement and Transport 79
   Distilled Water 80
   Water Intake Versus Water Output 82
   Water Therapy and Oncology 98

Chapter 6 - Oxygen, Ozone and Youthful Aging. 101
   The Oxidation Process 103
   Oxygen and Ozone 105

Chapter 7 - Impact of Stress 121
   Flight or Fight 127
   Stress Factors 129

Chapter 8 - Nutrition, Diet, and Supplements 139
   Nutrition and Diet 145
   Therapeutic Nutrition 148

Chapter 9 - Toxic Dentistry **159**
   Disease has its Origin in the Mouth! 160

Chapter 10 - Solutions to the Catastrophe **167**
   Humic Shale 168
   Fulvic Acid 171
   Growth and Maintenance Nutrients 178
   Nutritional Deficiencies 178
   The Vitamin Connection 180
   Free Radicals and Antioxidants 182
   Free Radical Scavengers 182
   Sea Minerals 185

Chapter 11 - The Potential of Personal Life Force 189

Appendix A - The Periodic Table **191**

Appendix B - Mineral Interaction Chart **201**

Appendix C - Mercury Exposure from Silver Tooth Fillings **209**

Appendix D - pH Saliva Test **225**

Appendix E - Amino Acids **229**
   Essential Amino Acids 230
   Enzymes 234

Glossary **236**

References and Recommended Reading **246**

About the Author **288**

Chapter 1
Introduction

This book aims to focus attention on the escalating catastrophe perpetuated by vested interest groups, ignored by government, and disastrous suppression of information, education and training regarding one of nature's most vital resources critical to the health of every individual on this planet.

We present evidence that the depletion of minerals in our soils, due to current destructive agricultural methods, produces deficient, chemicalized plant food. This depletion of minerals is a direct link to the escalating so called morbidity statistics of illness, disease and deaths that will continue to escalate causing more suffering and more serious diseases currently unimaginable.

Humankind has neglected the most important key to vibrant health that is the minerals and trace elements essential to a healthy balance in every cell in the body. This is clearly explained so as to understand the synergistic chemistry essential to the homeostasis involving the interaction between vitamins, amino acids and enzymes critical to good health.

We describe research experience relating to the critical pH balance dependent on the electrolyte chemistry presenting evidence that an alkaline pH is essential to vibrant health and that illness and disease develops in an acid pH.

We challenge the current approach presented by health experts, classifying fruit, vegetables and food as acid or alkaline as unscientific, followed by his interpretation of what causes acid pH and how to correct the problem.

This is not only about minerals, the electrolyte chemistry and pH. We presents information describing other factors that deplete mineral reserves including dehydration, inadequate oxygen, stress and infection as well as toxic dentistry. We suggest guidelines emphasizing that a program implementing all of these simultaneously, leads to the most successful outcome in the shortest possible time.

Morbidity Statistics

In the past year, more than 500,000 Americans died of heart disease and 600,000 died of cancer. Most of these deaths occurred in spite of the most advanced medical care available. Tragically, our medical system focuses on the development of new technology and methods to treat these diseases rather than a focus to understand and reveal the source or origin. The fact is that the increasing evidence as exampled in this book is that a substantial number of these deaths demonstrate a severe deficiency of essential minerals. In fact the scientific research demonstrates that when minerals are well supplied to maintain homeostasis of the electrolyte chemistry, these diseases do not occur.

Further, the scientific evidence demonstrates that even when heart disease, cancer and most degenerative disease are diagnosed, the successful restoration of this homeostatic electrolyte chemistry has the most potential to reverse these diseases.

This book reveals the extent of this problem, how this has occurred, the impact of minerals in health and disease, as well as information essential to ensure the correct choice and use of minerals to reverse illness and disease.

For those seeking vibrant health, this information describes how the correct choice and use of minerals electro-charge every cell in the body to achieve a vibrant health not possible with any other approach.

Youthful Life Extension

There is ample evidence that mankind is meant to live to ages 120 - 135. Over the years, well-known researchers have travelled the world to document with photographs cultures who live to be 135 years old and more, while retaining vibrant health and vigorous youth. Examples include the Japanese on Okinawa, Tibetans, the Hunzukuts of Northern Pakistan, the Armenian, the Georgians, the Azerbaijanis, the Vilcabamba Indians in Ecuador and the Titicacas in Peru.

Human Intervention

Generally the perception is that the earth is abundantly supplied with minerals. When pilgrims first landed in America more than 300 years ago, the average amount of topsoil was more than 3 feet deep. Today, it is estimated that only 6 inches remains.

Whereas early settlers moved from one growing area to another to benefit from fresh new growing and grazing, this trend changed to farming in permanent sites depleting the topsoil even further. The use of chemical phosphates to produce plants that appear to be healthy has resulted in unnatural depleted and chemicalized agricultured food.

In the year 1840 Professor Justus van Liebig published A the Organic Chemistry of Agriculture that led Chemical Companies to embrace his principle of supplying nitrogen, phosphorus and potassium (NPK) to unproductive soils, and began prospering with their artificial fertilizers in the late 19th century. These fertilizers made it possible for farmers to stop moving and stay in the same location - farming the same land indefinitely. The outcome of this early reliance on chemical fertilizers is the intensive chemical agriculture as we know it today.

The use of unnatural petrochemical fertilizers produced crops that looked healthy. However, the increasingly damaging effect of bugs able to attack weakened plant defense systems led to the use of pesticides. This combination of fertilizers and pesticides made it possible to obtain high yields of crops virtually free of insect damage. In the beginning results were impressive, but by the 1950's ever more potent chemicals had to be used to produce the same results. By 1960 farmers had already pumped 600 million pounds of chemicals into the soil and the food supply.

The use of pesticides continues unabated in spite of increasing reports of poisoning. A report published by the National Cancer Institute describes a study estimating that farm workers are six times more likely to contract cancer as compared to other non-agricultural workers. Data supplied by the National Academy of

Sciences reports 20,000 cases of cancer a year can be linked to pesticide poisoning.

The latest insult is the GMO (genetically modified organism), genetic engineering of seeds. It is not coincidental that chronic disorders like cancer, heart disease and other degenerative diseases have escalated since GMO food.

Studies have demonstrated that the application of chemicals to soil and plants has a direct relationship to ill health, death and the growing sensitivity to chemicals, food and atmospheric pollution.

The presence of chemical additives in food causes trace elements to become unavailable. The same applies to the soil trace elements that become unavailable to plants. Essential enzyme reactions are influenced by the shortage of any functional nutrient. Billions of microorganisms essential to the growth and health of the plant perish leading to sterile depleted soil.

Adding to this problem, the industrial revolution led to the refining and processing of staple food. Clearly, the depletion of essential nutrients corresponds to the escalating level of morbidity statistics of illness, disease and deaths that will continue to worsen unless we return to the soil those essential nutrients particularly minerals and trace elements.

Neglected Area of Research

The subject of the importance of minerals in health and disease is a neglected area of research - a subject as important as oxygen. In fact, the two work together. The same as the body cannot survive without oxygen, the body cannot survive without minerals. Various levels of depleted oxygen, as is the case for depleted minerals, determine the illness or diseases of mankind. Whereas the body can use food to produce energy and some vitamins, the body must have minerals supplied from plant source.

Although the evidence is overwhelming, and has been for a number years, giant agribusiness has successfully suppressed research that would demonstrate the relationship of chemical farming to illness and disease. Even a small percentage of the annual 750 million dollars currently spent on so called health care allocated to research would present evidence that could lead to the most dramatic change in our food supply to reverse the escalating suffering illness and deaths.

Importance of Minerals

Correctly described, minerals are electrolytes. Dr. Carey Reams, a biophysicist and biochemist determined that the body requires 84 of the known 106 elements to maintain optimum health. Many more than are currently recognized. Scientists estimate others have still to be revealed.

Each has a particular ionic charge that together is referred to as electrolytes. They have critical chemistry needed to balance heart rhythms, pH, body fluid, neurological transmission, and a myriad of cell molecular and atomic functions including structuring RNA characteristic of every cell.

When in balance vibrant health is obvious. When not in balance, a vast range of symptoms, illness and disease results. When illness and disease occur, the evidence is that the so-called miracle of healing is achieved when an imbalance of minerals is restored. On the other hand, failure to restore the mineral balance as we treat the symptoms, so we perpetuate the escalation of all our illness and disease.

Balancing Minerals

Before initiating the balancing of minerals, there are several factors that need to be understood to achieve success.

Inorganic Minerals

Inorganic minerals (metallic minerals) found in abundance in our soils and rocks are unnatural to the human body and can be toxic in this form.

Our creator intended that we get our minerals from plants grown in mineral rich soils. Plants absorb metallic minerals through their roots and convert them into organic hydrophilic minerals easily digested and assimilated. These plant minerals are hydrophilic or water soluble, which is what causes them to work efficiently with the natural body absorption and assimilation process.

Colloidal minerals have a negative electrical charge and each is hundreds of times smaller than a metallic mineral. Because of this negative charge and smaller size colloids stay in solution rather than going into suspension.

Several Forms of Minerals - Overview

There are different forms of minerals. Using the wrong kind of minerals can be toxic or fail to restore or maintain mineral balance. This is explained as follows:

Inorganic metallic minerals are those commonly used in the form of compressed tablets and are poorly used and more likely pass through the body without being digested. Even when dissolved in the digestive tract, the metallic salts which are positively charged ions are repelled by the positively charged lining of the digestive system leading to as little as 3-12% absorption.

There are supplements that have only 8-14 minerals whereas the body needs more than 74 to satisfy natural balance.

In the 1970's, the health food industry introduced chelated minerals to improve the absorption of minerals. This process uses an organic negatively charged amino acid molecule to bind with the positively charged metallic minerals. This larger negatively charged mineral compound is electrochemically attracted to the lining of the digestive tract and is thus more readily absorbed. However, the evidence is that the metallic mineral is inefficient in cell chemistry compared to natural plant minerals.

Then followed the introduction of plant derived minerals, in a colloidal solution. Colloidals are live energized nutrients which go to work immediately in cells throughout the body as compared to capsules and pills containing dried, desiccated and comatose nutrients requiring the body's energy and gastro-chemistry to initiate transport to the blood stream and thereafter to the cells. Colloidal formulations provide a more effective means of delivery, immediate absorption, and compatibility in body fluids.

1. Humic Shale

Chapter 2
A Review of Organic and Homeopathic Minerals

Extracted from a prehistoric petrified forest concentration of plant source and then combined with a colloidal solution. This extraction exposes these plant minerals to an unnatural process; considered necessary to produce plant derived minerals. When added to a colloidal solution this solution provides a more effective source of assimilable minerals.

2. Coral Calcium Powder

Supplies calcium and 75 trace minerals. Used by the Japanese living in the Okinawa Islands, who live beyond 100 years in great health, is attributed to coral powder.

Coral Calcium was first introduced to Western culture when it was brought to Europe by the Spanish explorers about 500 years ago who were amazed at the obvious vibrant health, energy and the number of centenarians on the islands. The world's oldest drugstores in Spain, which today are historic monuments, have clay pots on their shelves labeled Coral Calcium, Okinawa Japan. Literature written by doctors of the day told of miraculous cures. By the turn of the 20th Century, the consumption of coral had spread to mainland Japan, where currently there are about 17,000,000 users. Today there are millions of consumers in China, Russia, Britain, France and Sweden.

The success of coral calcium has unfortunately, also led to altered and polluted versions of the natural coral calcium that is described here so that our readers seek out the pure original natural powder form of this coral.

When coral calcium was brought to the Western communities as a modern dietary supplement in the 1970's, much misunderstanding was propagated by marketing companies. One example was the introduction of coral sand in tea bag form claiming to have the same benefits as powder. As a result there is a naive notion that when coral calcium is added to water it should dissolve completely. When asked about this, the answer is obvious. If coral were completely soluble in water there would be no coral reefs in the oceans!

The reason why this question is asked often relates to the popular use of coral sand in tea bags added to water as a tea. Coral calcium tea bags can impart desirable properties to water, such as the transfer of important marine microbes. A coral tea bag is about 2% of the marine nutrients that dissolve and the consumer, unless told, is almost unaware that they are consuming coral water, and not obtaining the full benefits of coral calcium when it is consumed in its complete form, supplying more than 50 times as much mineral nutrients. Also, the marine coral that is totally consumed is rich in all other nutrients.

Fossilized coral that has been washed up onto beaches has lost some of the mineral content by weathering and it may be dried and finely powdered to make a quick change of water pH. In addition, some commercially available coral calcium products have calcium added in hydroxide forms to increase alkalinity. Also, fossilized coral contains less than 1% magnesium, whereas marine coral has about 12% magnesium, which balances the 24% calcium for a perfect biological

2:1 calcium/magnesium ratio. Because of this lack of magnesium in fossilized coral, magnesium compounds are often added, resulting in a substantial dilution of the coral. After study of many types of coral supplements, the evidence clearly demonstrates that marine coral, not fossilized coral, taken in complete form is obviously the most ideal way to consume coral calcium.

As a result of competition, those selling fossilized coral mislead the public into thinking that because they remove their coral from beaches they are not harming the coral reefs, implying that those mining the marine coral must be harming the reefs. The truth is that the harvesting of the marine coral is done under the strict supervision of the Japanese Government who enforces regulations and incarcerate violators if the slightest damage occurs. In reality, the deposition of the coral sands (coral calcium) at the base of the reef actually inhibits the growth of the coral reefs. The islands of Okinawa are very shallow with little wave action allowing the coral sands to pile up, choking off the reef. In places like Hawaii, where there is lots of wave action, the coral sands get washed out into the ocean. When the coral sands are removed by harvesting, the reefs come alive and flourish. Thus harvesting marine coral calcium is not only beneficial to man but to the coral reefs as well.

Many commercial companies have promoted coral calcium from Okinawa as though it is all the same material. However, the harvesting of marine bed coral is much more difficult and costly than merely collecting fossilized coral from beach mines. This fossilized coral has undergone thousands, if not millions, of years of erosion. Losing most of its magnesium content and much of its trace metal content.

Also, because of the hype generated by coral calcium testimonials, numerous, unscrupulous entrepreneurs are harvesting coral from other locations around the world (such coral does not have the desired microbes), but telling their customers that it comes from Okinawa. Some even go so far as to blend their coral with Okinawa coral so that they can make the claim that it comes from Okinawa.

In studies of the selection of different types of coral, it has been learned that careful selection of suitable grade material is essential. Therefore it is shocking to find that some commercial types of coral calcium are less than 10% coral calcium.

This practice has emerged in the manufacture of types of coral calcium capsules. The addition of inert magnesium or calcium should be disclosed by manufacturers on their labels. A label that declares a minimum of 1000 milligrams of coral calcium content from Okinawa in a daily dose, preferably marine coral, is acceptable. Many of the diluted versions have less than 500 milligrams of coral calcium per daily dose.

As mentioned earlier, marine based or fossilized coral calcium does not provide the amount of magnesium to meet recommended levels for health. This is why nutrition with high magnesium and mineral diets are an important factor in health maintenance. After all the term dietary supplement must be understood that supplements are not to be confused as alternatives to a healthy balanced diet. The word supplement implies extra nutrient ingredients to provide health benefits over and above a balanced diet.

Despite the deficiencies, both tea bag coral and fossilized coral consumption have led to remarkable health testimonials, although not as many as the consumption of marine coral. This is due to the presence of the microbe factor. In addition there are many other factors that make coral calcium of marine origin more ideal for health. The use of vegetable capsules or at least capsules that are made to dissolve at the right time to provide the best circumstances for mineral absorption is preferable. The practice of breaking capsules and adding the contents to water is unnecessary, except in circumstances where some people cannot swallow capsules.

The author recommends a specific Okinawa coral calcium powder from an approved supplier complying with the best quality standards of selection and packaging.

About Coral Reefs

Coral reefs are an example of one of natures creations that deserves description here. Coral reefs are sea mountains of minerals of which calcium predominates, along with numerous other inorganic and organic forms of calcium. In order to build a reef, the living coral polyps require specific climatic and ecological conditions. Indeed, coral reefs are most preponderant in warm shallow waters of the ocean, which have a range of temperature from approximately 20⁰C centigrade) to 30⁰C.

Without sunlight the living infrastructure of organisms on the reef that use photosynthesis for nutrition cannot survive. These photosynthetic organisms, algae, are quite primitive, but efficient in forming a basic nutrient source for the food chain of reef dwellers. Some marine organisms rely heavily on the photosynthesizing organisms. The most interesting aspect of coral is their efficient and versatile ability to reproduce. They can reproduce by budding in an asexual manner and many polyps can form with remaining connections to its forerunner. Once a year, the corals may spawn filling areas of the reef with massive amounts of eggs and sperm (the reefs are submerged in a cloud of sperm and eggs) which attract plankton eating fish and mammals.

The basic photosynthetic organisms and plant life provide food for vegetarian inhabitants such as damsel fish, parrot fish, blennies and puffer fish. The parrot fish play a unique role in the biomass of reefs. They use their strong teeth to chew coral which is ground-up in their digestive tract and released to form the sandy base of the reef. In fact, parrot fish and similar coral munchers are a prime source of marine coral that is harvested as coral calcium.

It is clear that the geological evolution of Okinawa and its adjacent islands affects the environmental availability of minerals. The islands are composed of about 60 land masses of variable size that form an arc in the ocean, spanning several hundred miles. The largest land masses are volcanic in origin with raised profiles, but coral islands tend to be flat. A unique feature of this geography that may account for even more abundance of various minerals, is the proximity of coral reefs to volcanic material. Volcanic material forms soils that are exceedingly rich in trace elements, resulting in an even greater source of minerals that are incorporated into Okinawa coral. Thus the coral from Okinawa is dramatically chemically different from all other coral. In addition, its marine microbes are specific to the islands of Okinawa, and are not found in other coral, thus it is uniquely different from all other coral.

Sea Minerals Formula

Included here is a unique formula containing minerals derived from sea plants in combination with plant extracts of enzymes, amino acids, vitamins plus aloe and Pau DArco. This book has explained the importance of synergistic nutrients working together with minerals to achieve a homeostasis to maximize vibrant health. This sea plant mineral formula is a unique balance of essential minerals, amino acids, vitamins and enzymes in a colloid solution.

Sea minerals are uniquely identical to those in the human body ensuring 95-98% absorption. The manufacturer claims to have achieved a similar absorption factor for all the ingredients in the formula. They claim to use appropriate methods of farming techniques utilizing seaweed and microorganisms for fertilization to increase the nutritional qualities to very high levels. It is grown and harvested only when ripe, from the coldest and purest seawater from around the world. They claim the formula is approximately 50 times more potent in nutritional value than sea kelp!

The author recommends this formula as a baseline to which one or more of the other mineral formulae is added depending on individual health or illness and disease. For example coral calcium has a different biochemistry to the homeopathic formula of minerals described in this section.

As has been described, sea minerals are found to be the closest to that found in the human body. Our more advanced understanding of the chemistry emphasizes the critical synergistic interaction with other nutrients, vitamins, amino acids and enzymes. Clearly, the ultimate daily diet should provide pollution and chemically free organically grown food in nutrient rich soils. Scientists continue to research and attempt to develop a natural supplement formula to compare with this ultimate diet and nutrition without success - a challenge most unlikely to duplicate nature. However, the author is of the opinion that one sea mineral based complete formula available as a supplement has achieved a balance using a sea plant source to deliver a true synergistic formula combining minerals, vitamins, amino acids and enzymes, a breakdown which is presented here as follows:

> INGREDIENTS: Matrix Aloe Vera Proprietary process Aloe vera barbadensis Miller (whole inner leaf) Sealogica Proprietary Sea-Veg Blend Alaria Esculenta Costaria Costata Enteromorpha Linza Fucus Gardneri Fucus Vesiculosus Gigartina Alveata Laminaria Digitata Nereocystis Luetkeana Rhodymenia Pertusa Ulva Latuca Phyto-Silver Pau D'Arco Extract (Quadruple Strength) Tabebuia impetiginosa (inner bark) Natural Cranberry Matrix Aloe Vera and Sealogica

TRACE MINERALS: Barium Bismuth Boron Bromine Cadmium Caesium Cerium Chloride Chromium Cobalt Copper Fluorine Gallium Germanium Gold Indium Iodine Iron Iridium Lanthanum Lithium Manganese Molybdenum Nickel Niobium Osmium Palladium Platinum Rhodium Rubidium Selenium Silica Silicon Strontium Silver Sodium Sulfur Tellurium Tin Titanium Tungsten Uranium Vanadium Zinc Zirconium

BIO-ELEMENTS	ENZYMES
Carbon Hydrogen Nitrogen Oxygen	Amylase Cellulase Lipase Protease

Homeopathic Formula

In addition to the above, there is also a homeopathic formula developed by a naturopathic physician based on the earlier work of Dr. George H. Earp-Thomas.

In the 1930's, Earp-Thomas discovered that without minerals, cells can not maintain cell wall pressure (osmotic equilibrium) become weak and susceptible to infection and disease. This insight inspired his careful study of how minerals become biologically available. He began to devise natural methods to deliver minerals to cells as electrolytes in biological not merely chemical form.

Earp-Thomas worked on the electrolyte formula diligently. He determined which elements were compatible in a homeopathic formula, not by guesswork, but by observing mineral uptake in wheat grass he grew organically on his farm. Patient trial and error, and careful observation of many repetitious experiments continued for several years.

By 1938, he had a crude stage of electrolyte solution using a three- phase process: water, bacteria and electromagnetic spin.

Subsequent development led to liquid crystalloid electrolytes far beyond minerals. In a biological method of production, over the course of a week in a vat, minerals are transformed into a special state by bacteria, and acquire an added energy force. If you try to measure it, its not detectable.

This force is not a mystery, but is subtle beyond mans most sensitive instruments.

The best way to describe this state is that minerals change form to become energized like plasma - a living water, in complex, stable, yet changing states of charge.

In fact, by coincidence, the medical term for the fluid in blood is plasma. In physics plasma is the fourth state of matter - an ionized, electrified state.

Added to pure water (three stages beyond distillation) carefully measured mineral salts: two major elements - sodium and potassium - in parts per thousand with nine trace elements -copper, iodine, manganese, zinc, cobalt, selenium, chromium, silica, and boron, in parts per million or less.

Minerals must be super-pure as there can be no contamination with other elements, or electrolytes wont form; proportion is more critical than amount.

Measuring must be precise. Minerals are measured down to exact micrograms, and cannot be off by a hair or they won't go into solution, but drop to the bottom of the tank.

Only certain minerals will form these electrolytes. There is no iron in the formula. This essential mineral wont form electrolytes - maybe cobalt is a precursor. Drinking electrolytes creates an electromagnetic energy in the body that will pull iron from food - and out of the blood, into cells. Iron is magnetic. In this condition, the minerals are so dilute it is like pure drinking water.

They are as essential as carbohydrates and protein, but needed in minute amounts. For example, we need little more than a millionth of an ounce of iodine, but if it is lacking, goiter develops from a dysfunctional thyroid.

A cell wall cannot have elasticity unless it has a minute trace of silica. As we get older, lack of silica causes skin to harden and age rapidly. With silica, skin stays younger. Silica is the cement that holds bone together.

Combining these elements is a sensitive challenge, since minerals have complex interactions with each other and other nutrients. Some are beneficial, but many are antagonistic. For example, zinc interferes with copper and iron absorption, while copper enhances iron uptake, but inhibits molybdenum. Cobalt is antagonized by molybdenum, and unfriendly to zinc.

The challenge requires the right minerals at the right times on the right days in the right quantities. The ratios of the elements are more important than actual amounts. If the ratios are not there, electrolytes wont form properly.

Minerals in the homeopathic formula are beyond a dissolved state. They are energized by living biological process. To the carefully prepared solution a common bacteria is added - this is what makes it come alive - a wonderful, fascinating process as nature creating life itself.

Bacteria feed on the minerals, change them from simple ionic solution to an electromagnetic state of charge similar to plasma - the fourth state of matter. While this metamorphosis is no mystery, it is subtle and obscure beyond the means and models of modern science.

This homeopathic crystalloid mineral is now used by an increasing number of enlightened individuals who report dramatic improvement in health.

Chapter 3
Overview of Minerals And Trace Elements

It has been suggested that "99% of American people are deficient in minerals. A marked deficiency in any one or more of the important minerals actually results in disease." U.S. Senate Document #264

This introduction preceding the following list describing minerals is necessarily technical in some of the cell chemistry. It is particularly important to present an overview of the synergistic chemistry of minerals with vitamins, amino acids and enzymes. Like an orchestra of 80 musicians, when each is in harmony the symphony is dynamic and beautiful. When one or more are not in tune, the result is discord and collapse. On the other hand, reestablishing balance to the weak players will return harmony to the symphony.

Macro and Micro-Minerals

The essential macro-minerals, that is, minerals required in dietary amounts of 100mg per day or more, include calcium, phosphorus, sodium, potassium, chlorine, magnesium, and sulfur.

Micro-minerals which are needed in quantities of

only a few milligrams or micrograms each day are iron, copper, cobalt, zinc, manganese, iodine, molybdenum, selenium, fluorine and chromium.

Nonessential contaminants include lead, cadmium, mercury, arsenic, barium, strontium, boron, aluminum, lithium, beryllium, rubidium, as well as others not listed here. (Boron, lithium and rubidium are used in treatment of certain types of disease).

Although the essential micro-minerals consist of only a minute fraction of the total body weight compared to the macro-minerals, their function is needed to produce energy, in growth and maintenance of body tissue, and the regulation of body processes indispensable to life processes cannot be over emphasized.

Continued ingestion of diets, or continued exposure to total environments that are deficient, polluted, imbalanced, or excessively high in a particular trace element, induces changes in the functioning forms, activities, or concentrations of that element in body tissues and fluids so that they fall below or rise above acceptable limits.

If the physiological role of food is to provide essential nutrients for normal functioning of the body, then a nutrient is a required substance that the body must obtain externally because it cannot manufacture that nutrient or in some cases cannot synthesize it at a sufficient rate to meet the bodys needs.

Energy is derived from carbohydrates, fats, and protein. Actual energy is obtained only upon oxidation of the energy nutrients. Vitamins and minerals primarily role is in the oxidation process as enzymatic cofactors.

Their role, and to a lesser extent the role of protein in the enzyme molecule, are indirect rather than directly contributing to the energy supply.

A second function is the growth and maintenance of body tissues. The principal structured materials of the body are water, protein and minerals. Some lipid-containing compounds are also found in the cell membranes. Vitamins do not directly contribute to physical body structure. Nevertheless, growth and maintenance of body tissues is impossible without them. For example, vitamin A does not appear to be in structural requirements of the retina of the eye per se, but without it the formation of the retina would not occur. The major role of the vitamins as a whole is as co-factors of specific enzymes.

Functioning as an enzymatic co-factor or activator is also an equally important role of minerals. For building protein tissues the different proteins that are ingested are not completely interchangeable. They must be digested into amino acids enzymatically and by changes in pH, before they can be restructured into new proteins. Many of the enzymes involved in these processes require specific minerals as activators or co-enzymes.

All of the nutrients - protein, carbohydrates, lipids, minerals, vitamins and water - help regulate body processes. Each nutrient by itself, or more generally in conjunction with other nutrients, perform certain functions that are essential to the normal body metabolism. For example, these include movement of fluids, control of the acid-base balance in the body, coagulation of blood, the activation of enzymes (to carry these as well as the other two basic functions of the nutrients above), and the maintenance of normal body temperatures, etcetera.

It should be remembered that an individual nutrient, such as a mineral, may fulfill all three of these functions. For example calcium is absolutely essential for the growth and maintenance of ossa (bone). The amount of calcium required for this bone growth varies with skeletal development, but even at the adult state, dietary calcium is constantly required to replace dissolved bone for skeletal maintenance.

Not only is calcium involved in the growth and maintenance of body tissue, but also the same metal regulates certain body functions. When a nerve impulse arrives at a neuromuscular junction acetylcholine is released.

Calcium and Electrical Nerve Impulse

Acetylcholine is involved in several enzymatic reactions that change the permeability of the nerve cell membranes. When this happens, $Na^%$ (symbol for the element sodium) and $K^%$ (symbol for the element potassium) move through the membrane creating an electrical impulse. This makes it possible for the nerve impulse to pass to the muscle. Calcium promotes the release of the acetylcholine and the sliding process of muscle contraction.

The stimulus that produces muscle contraction is an electrical impulse delivered by the motor nerve to the muscle cell. It travels along the membrane of the muscle fiber. The electrical activity increases the permeability of the membranes of the sarcoplasmic reticulum to calcium ions. The ions pour into cytoplasm, activating the troponin contractile mechanism. Troponin inhibits muscle contraction by blocking the interaction of the proteins action and myosin unless it is combined with calcium.

After contraction, calcium is quickly removed and returned to the storage sacs in the sarcoplasmic reticulum, and the muscle relaxes.

Potassium, sodium, and magnesium are also essential components in the muscle contraction-relaxation process.

The same mineral that is part of the bone structure and used to regulate body processes is also necessary for the production of energy in the body.

Calcium and Pancreatic Lipase

Calcium is absolutely necessary to activate the fat-splitting enzyme, pancreatic lipase. The cells of the pancreas that secrete insulin must have calcium in the intercellular fluid before they can respond to the stimulation from glucose.

Enzymes are extremely important when considering the function of minerals because the major role of the metals in carrying out their three functions is related to their various roles as co-factors or as influences on the enzymes. Through catalytic action, enzymes promote and regulate the multitude of chemical reactions essential for life within the organism.

Enzymes and Amino Acids

As an organic catalyst which facilitates specific reactions, enzymes are manufactured by cellular protoplasm and are either secreted into the body fluids or are produced and used within the cytoplasm of the body cells themselves.

It is estimated that the average cell contains several thousand different enzymes. Enzymes are proteins (polymers) composed of long chains of relatively low molecular weight amino acids. These amino acids contain both the alkaline amino (NH) group and the acidic carboxyl (COOH) group. This type of structure allows other compounds to be linked to these chains of amino acids through the process of chelation.

Chelated Amino Acids

Chelation of metal ions by integral proteins or with amino acids prior to ingestion is fundamental to their absorption from the gut. The metals are not absorbed or metabolized as isolated ions, but instead bonded to organic molecules.

Chelation occurs when more than one donor atom in a chelating agent, called the ligand, bonds to the metal ion through coordinate covalent bonds to form a ring-like molecule. Where the metal is bonded by two atoms in the same ligand molecule, a double heterocyclic ring structure may result. When both ligands are single amino acids, a dipeptide-like chelate is formed.

Many enzymes are more than simple proteins. Through chelation these specific complex proteins are linked to non-proteinaceous substances called prosthetic groups containing either a vitamin or a mineral. When the prosthetic group is part of the enzyme, the enzyme is called a metalloenzyme. When the prosthetic group is readily removed from the enzyme, it is called a cofactor. In this case, through chelation or complexing, a simple ion is attached to the protein and activates the enzyme. When the ion is removed from the enzyme, all of its catalytic ability is lost.

In Eichhorns discussion of enzymes he indicates that if the metal is weakly bonded to the protein, the ion may participate in bond cleavage reactions by altering the enzymes structure by pulling away the negative charge from the substrate and then attaching the enzyme to the substrate. If the metal is strongly bound to the protein molecule of the enzyme, then the ion participates in an electron transfer type of reaction. The catalytic activity of the enzyme is determined by how the protein is attached to the prosthetic group and the electronic configuration of the metal in the prosthetic group.

The cell is basically a metal deficiency system in which all of the ligands, including those forming enzymes, are in competition for a limited number of metal ions.

It is because they are essential components of certain enzyme systems that minerals play such an important role in biological processing, that deficiencies or excesses of them can seriously alter the enzymatic equilibrium of cells.

In summary, it has been seen that man and animals are autonomously functioning complex units whose basic structure is composed of carbon, hydrogen, oxygen, and nitrogen. In addition to these basic elements, living cells also require the macro-minerals sulfur, phosphorous, sodium, potassium, chlorine, calcium and magnesium. They are basic to the composition of the body. Finally, to complete the life processes, trace minerals are required for many vital functions. The great majority of the trace elements serve as key components of enzymatic systems or in proteins with other vital roles. Although the macro-minerals chief role is structural, they too can function in enzymes or in proteins. Many clinical and pathological disorders arise as a consequence of mineral deficiencies and/or excess.

This illustrates the numerous roles and interrelationship of minerals in nutrition, in health, and in disease and underline the importance of optimum mineral nutrition.

The following is a list of minerals and trace elements describing specific properties illustrating their essential role in the chemistry of the human body.

Magnesium

Best food sources of magnesium are whole grains and legumes. Over 80% of magnesium in grains is lost in the removal of the germ and outer layers of grains to make refined white and so-called enriched flour.

With the progressive degradation of our food, magnesium intake has progressively declined in developed countries. Our average daily intake is now only 329mg for males and 207mg for females, well below the RDA of 350mg and 280mg respectively (considered to be marginal).

Magnesium is the second most common mineral in the body and perhaps the fifth major nutrient of green plants. It is also the most overlooked and under-rated element of all by the medical, dental, veterinary and agricultural scientists, who tend to insist that there is so much magnesium about that it is not likely to be a problem. Their flimsy argument is that since the chlorophyll of all green plants contains magnesium then obviously there is no shortage.

There is a steady loss of magnesium due to the continued and injudicious use of NPK (super phosphates) chemical fertilizers, which in turn has given rise to an increasing number of metabolic disorders in both animals and human beings.

Here is a truth so incredible, as to be unbelievable. What has killed more Americans in the last 57 years than all American deaths in the war in Vietnam, Hitlers holocaust, and Hiroshima/Nagasaki atomic bombings combined? The gross deficiency of one single mineral in our diets! Magnesium!

Several groups in the United States are now compiling statistics and data, revealing what is becoming known as the Magnesium Catastrophe. Based on studies done in Canada, Finland, Great Britain and India, a global pattern of magnesium deficiency deaths has emerged. Estimates of annual U.S. deaths range from 215,000 to 869,000. Until recently, because of the implications, this information has been successfully kept from the public.

The U.S. Department of Agriculture reported that only 25% of 37,000 consumers surveyed had a dietary magnesium intake that equaled or exceeded the RDA (Recommended Daily Allowance), and this assumed their food had a normal concentration of magnesium!

Magnesium deficiency, without warning, causes cardiac disease, arrhythmia, cardiac death (heart attack) and more. It's unbelievable, but this is actually happening now!

In the American Journal of Surgery, four Medical Doctors reported investigations on magnesium therapy in bypass operations for the grossly obese. They discovered that with reduced absorption in the small intestine, and lowered magnesium intake, magnesium supplements were necessary to arrest serious and rapid deterioration of the health of the patient.

Dr. Kenneth Cooper, founder of the Dallas Aerobic Institute where the heart and lungs of athletes under stress are investigated, has suggested that cardiac arrhythmia — sudden death — is induced by nothing more than a temporary magnesium shortage. He now prescribes two dolomite tablets twice a day for his athletes after finding that West Coast distance runners had long been ingesting dolomite tablets as insurance against cramps.

Supporting this theory, Drs Burch and Giles from the Tulane University School of medicine in 1978 reported in the American Heart Journal, on Magnesium Deficiency in Cardiovascular Disease, that chronic low-grade magnesium deficiency may be much more common than is conventionally considered, since magnesium is not studied regularly in clinical medicine and that magnesium deficiency will be found only when looked for and thus responsibility for prevention, detection and treatment resides with the physician.

Back in 1957, Drs M. Shapiro and I. Bersohn of the Johannesburg Institute of Medical Research in South Africa, were involved in a study with spectacular results of magnesium therapy versus anticoagulant drugs (such as warfarin which is also used as a rat poison). This study was done on a large number of patients admitted to hospital with coronary thrombosis.

In their findings they stated: In one year 196 patients were admitted with severe coronary heart disease and were treated with normally accepted anticoagulants. 60 died.

In the following year over 100 patients were admitted with similar coronary complaints and were treated with intravenously administered magnesium. 1 died (British Medical Journal, 23 January 1960).

It is hard to believe that with such findings highlighting the role of magnesium in the immediate reduction of heart disease and reduction of cholesterol, the need for more magnesium in the diet has not been widely publicized. Worst still, if you were to study the contents of refined, processed food you will find that food technologists are not paying any attention to supplementation with magnesium in food contents.

Supplementation with magnesium as part of a complete mineral supplement is the only way to overcome this problem. 400-1200mg per day of magnesium can be used. If the colloidal form is not available then the aspartate form should be used. If the kidneys are healthy, there is no evidence of toxicity up to 6000mg per day.

Magnesium is an essential mineral accounting for about 0.05% of the body's total weight. Magnesium is involved in many essential metabolic processes.

1. Most magnesium is found inside the cell, where it activates enzymes necessary for the metabolism of carbohydrates and amino acids.

2. By countering the stimulative effect of calcium, magnesium plays an important role in neuromuscular contractions.

3. Magnesium helps regulate the acid-alkaline balance in the body.

4. Magnesium helps promote absorption and metabolism of other minerals such as calcium, phosphorus, sodium and potassium.
5. It also helps utilize the B Complex and Vitamins C and E in the body.
6. It aids bone growth.
7. Is necessary for proper functioning of the muscles including those of the heart.

The body contains only 20-30 grams of magnesium, about an ounce. It forms part of over 300 vital enzymes as well as part of bones.

Magnesium is essential to burn glycogen for fuel, muscle contraction, and transmission of the genetic code to form new proteins. It is needed to balance pH, assists in calcium and potassium assimilation.

It is also a key mineral for heart health. It is also the key mineral in carbohydrate and mineral metabolism.

Magnesium may be beneficial for the following ailments: Arteriosclerosis, Atherosclerosis, High Cholesterol Level, Diabetes, Hypertension, High LDL Cholesterol, Fracture, Osteoporosis, Rickets, Colitis, Diarrhea, Depression, Epilepsy, Mental Illness, Multiple Sclerosis, Nervousness, Neuritis, Neuromuscular Disorders, Noise Sensitivity, Parkinson's Disease, Tantrums, Hand Tremors, Coronary Thrombosis, Ischemic Heart Disease, Celiac Disease, Arthritis, Kidney Stones, Oxalate Stones, Leg Cramps, Muscle Weakness, Muscular Excitability, Neuromuscular Disorders, Weakness, Psoriasis, Decay, Vomiting, Alcoholism, Backache, Convulsions, Delirium, Epilepsy, Kwashiorkor, Overweight, Obesity, PMS, and Polio.

Calcium

Calcium is the most abundant mineral in the body and the fifth most abundant substance. About 99% is deposited in the bones and teeth.

The remaining 1% is involved in the soft tissues, intracellular fluids and blood.

A major function of calcium is to act synergistically with phosphorus to build and maintain healthy bones and teeth.

Another important function is storage of the mineral in the bones for use by the body. The calcium state of the bones is constantly fluctuating according to the diet and to the body's needs.

The 1% of ionized calcium that circulates in the fluids of the body is small, but vital to life.

a) It is essential for healthy blood.

b) Eases insomnia.

c) Its delicate messenger ions help regulate the heartbeat. Along with calcium, magnesium is needed to properly maintain the cardiovascular system. In addition calcium assists in the process of blood clotting. Helps prevent the accumulation of too much acid or too much alkali in the blood.

d) It plays a part in secretion of hormones.

e) It affects neurotransmitters (serotonin, acetylcholine and norepinephrine), nerve transmission, muscle growth and muscle contraction.

f) The mineral acts as a messenger from the cell surface to the inside of the cell and helps regulate the passage of nutrients in and out of the cell walls.

g) A body of 70kg contains about 1.3kg of calcium, 99% of it in the bones and teeth. The other 1% flows in and out of cells controlling conduction of impulses in nerves, contraction of muscles, and many other functions essential to continuing life. So whenever this vital 1% of calcium is not supplied by nutrition, even for one day, the body cannibalizes (eats up) its own bones to make up the deficit.

Milk -only raw organic whole full cream milk should be used. The cream is high in vitamin A and is needed for calcium metabolism. Cooking, pasteurizing and homogenizing destroys vitamins and enzymes and alters the protein. Powdered milk (even spray-dried) is cooked. It is also high in artificial vitamin D and quite high in strontium. A cup or two a day could be toxic. A large glass of raw, whole cream organic milk contains about 500mg of calcium. Of that, 150mg is absorbed.

Pasteurized, homogenized low fat milk is not a well tolerated food for adults or children, and, because of our degraded food and dietary habits, average intake of calcium in America is only around 750mg per day. Thats way below the top RDA of 1200mg. Other good sources of dietary calcium include; dried figs, sardines, sesame seed, and green leafy vegetables.

Apart from people with a tendency to form calcium oxalate (kidney stones), calcium is non-toxic to at least 2500mg per day. Supplements of 400-1600mg can be used daily. Apart from colloidal form, calcium citrate and calcium carbonate are good forms, with excellent absorption rates. Avoid bone meal, however, which is contaminated with lead. If mineral supplements are to be taken once a day, then it is suggested they are taken at night, because the mineral flux in the body that maintains bone growth is greatest during sleep.

Calcium deficiency has been indicated with the following ailments: Anemia, Diabetes, Hemophilia, Pernicious Anemia, Backache, Fracture, Osteomalacia, Osteoporosis, Rickets, Colitis, Diarrhea, Dizziness, Epilepsy, Finger Tremors, Insomnia, Irritability, Mental Illness, Nervousness, Parkinson's Disease, Meniere's Syndrome, Cataracts, Headache, Arteriosclerosis, Atherosclerosis, Hypertension, High LDL Levels, Cancer of the Large Intestine, Celiac Disease, Constipation, Hemorrhoids, Worms, Arthritis, Rheumatism, Nephritis, Muscle Cramps, Allergies, Common Cold, Tuberculosis, Tetany, Nail Problems, Acne, Bee and Spider Bites, Sunburn, Stomach Ulcers, Brittle Teeth, Cavities, Pyorrhea, Tooth and Gum Disorders, Aging Fever, Overweight, Obesity, and Toxicity.

Phosphorus

The body has about 800 grams of phosphorus, 700 grams in the bones. The other 100 grams is essential for a multitude of purposes, from the energy cycle, to the formation of red blood cells.

Phosphorus is everywhere in food and more is added during food processing. Best sources are meat, milk, fish and whole grains. Average daily intake is about 1500mg for males, and 1000mg for females so deficiency is rare. Instead, because of food processing, there is a phosphorus overload.

Phosphorus is found in every cell and is one of the most abundant minerals in the body. A balance of calcium and phosphorus is needed to be effectively used by the body. Because it is in every cell, phosphorus plays a part in almost every chemical reaction within the body.

It is important in the utilization of carbohydrates, fats and protein for growth, maintenance and repair, both within and outside of the cells, and for the production of energy.

It stimulates muscle contractions, including the regular contractions of the heart muscle.

Niacin and riboflavin cannot be digested unless phosphorus is present.

Phosphorus is an essential part of nucleoproteins, which are responsible for cell division and reproduction.

Phosphorus helps prevent the accumulation of too much acid or too much alkali in the blood, assists in the passage of substances through the cell walls and promotes the secretion of glandular hormones.

It is also needed for healthy nerves and efficient mental activity.

B-Complex vitamins and many enzymes require phosphorus to function.

Phosphorus may be beneficial for the following ailments: Fractures, Osteomalacia, Osteoporosis, Rickets, Stunted Growth, Colitis, Mental Illness, Mental Stress, Arteriosclerosis, Atherosclerosis, Arthritis, Arthritic Conditions, Leg Cramps, Tooth and Gum Disorders, Alcoholism, Backache, Cancer Prevention, Pregnancy and Stress.

Potassium

Good food sources of potassium are bananas and green leafy vegetable. Most fresh food, even fish, is high in potassium and low sodium. The average ratio of potassium to sodium is 7:1 in a mixed fresh food diet. Added sodium during processing reverses these ratios to 3.5 part sodium to 1 part potassium, leading to excess sodium and a deficiency in potassium.

Average potassium intake has fallen to 2500mg per day, and much of that is lost again in people who use antibiotics or diuretics. The official recommended intake is 3500mg per day.

Supplements of 100-500mg per day are preferably in the aspartate form if colloidal minerals cannot be obtained. Potassium is not toxic up to about 5000mg per day, but if taken without food it can burn and upset the gut.

Potassium is an essential mineral found mainly in the intracellular fluid (98%), where it is the primary positive ion force.

Potassium constitutes 5% of the total mineral content of the body and preserves proper alkalinity of the body fluids.

Potassium and sodium help regulate water balance within the body, that is, they help regulate the distribution of fluids on either side of the cell walls. Potassium also regulates the transfer of nutrients to the cells.

Potassium combines with phosphorus to send oxygen to the brain and functions with calcium in the regulation of neuromuscular activity.

The synthesis of muscle protein and protein from the amino acids in the blood requires potassium.

Protein and carbohydrate metabolism is dependent upon potassium. It stimulates the kidneys to eliminate poisonous body wastes.

Potassium works with sodium to help normalize the heartbeat. Potassium is the main cation (positively charged electrolyte) inside cells. It interacts with sodium and chloride in conduction of nerve impulses and a host of other duties.

Potassium may be beneficial for the following ailments: Angina, Pectoris, Diabetes, Hypertension, Hypoglycemia, Hypoglycemia, Mononucleosis, Stroke, Fracture, Colitis, Diarrhea, Alcoholism, Insomnia, Poor Reflexes, Polio, Fever, Headache, Congestive Heart Failure, Myocardial Infarction, Constipation, Worms, Arthritis, Gout, Allergies, Impaired Muscle Activity, Muscular Dystrophy, Rheumatism, Sterility, Acne, Burns, Dermatitis, Colic Gastroenteritis, Tooth and Gum Disorders, Cancer, Impaired Growth and Stress.

Trace Minerals

Boron

Boron occurs widely in food in trace amounts, especially in soybeans, prunes, raisins, almonds and dates. Average daily intake is about 1.9mg.

There are reports that because of their greater hormone demands, athletes are supplemented with 3-6mg of boron daily in mixed citrate and aspartate forms, all other patients use the colloidal form.

Boron is a low toxicity mineral, but intake above 50mg per day can interfere with phosphorus and riboflavin metabolism.

Boron -a) Reduces calcium loss from bones. b) Boron was recently shown to be essential for the manufacture of some hormones. c) Despite the hype of some supplement makers, however, boron is not anabolic, that is, does not cause muscle growth. Nor does it increase testosterone levels.

Cesium

Enters cancer cells and produces alkaline condition, causing cancer cells to die.

Chloride

Chloride is the main anion (negatively charged electrolyte) outside cells. It works with sodium and potassium to regulate fluid and electrolyte balance.

Chloride is an essential mineral occurring in the body mainly in compound form with sodium or potassium.

Along with our excessive sodium in salt added to our food, we also get excessive chloride from other sources - about 6 grams daily, whereas we need less than one gram daily. However, a low salt diet equals low sodium and low chloride intake, a wise dietary strategy.

Chromium

This mineral is important in carbohydrate metabolism. Organic chromium is an active ingredient of a substance called GTF (glucose tolerance factor); niacin and amino acids complete the formula.

Chromium stimulates the activity of enzymes involved in the metabolism of glucose for energy and the synthesis of fatty acids and cholesterol.

It appears to increase the effectiveness of insulin and its ability to handle glucose, preventing hypoglycemia or diabetes. Chromium is essential for glucose, insulin, fatty acid, and protein metabolism.

Best sources of chromium are whole grains and shellfish, but up to 90% of chromium is lost in food processing. Because of our food degradation, chromium is one of the most frequently deficient minerals in the Western diet. Average daily intake of chromium is only 2533mcg. The American RDA handbook recommends 50-200mcg per day. So supplementation is essential for optimal health.

200-800mcg per day of chromium have been used for athletes.

The best form is chromium picolinate. Although developed in early 80s, chromium picolinate now has more than 40 research studies showing that it improves insulin metabolism, reduces body fat, increases lean muscle, and lowers cholesterol.

Chromium picolinate shows no toxicity in amounts of 10-50mg. This may not apply to other forms of chromium.

For normal routine prevention supplementation, the colloidal form twice a day is preferable to ensure that sudden GTF (glucose tolerance factor) problems do not drain energy.

Cobalt

Cobalt is an integral part of vitamin B12. Cobalt acts as a substitute for manganese in activating a number of enzymes in the body. It replaces zinc in some enzymes and activates others as well.

It is necessary for normal functioning and maintenance of red blood cells, as well as all other body cells.

Cobalt is present in ocean and sea vegetation, but is lacking in almost all land grown, green food.

Vegetables can grow well in the absence of cobalt in the soil. It has not been proven that plants need cobalt at all. However, vegetables are a vehicle for cobalt to enter our own bodies, and for vegetarians no cobalt in the soil means no cobalamin (vitamin B12), resulting in pernicious anemia.

This problem does not arise with meat eaters, for meat is rich in cobalt.

Copper

Copper is an excellent catalyst for oxidation-reduction systems, showing great versatility for an impressive variety of reactions, including the formation of water from oxygen and hydrogen at body temperatures; this reaction would be explosive without copper. It is an unique agent in biological systems, all living things require it, and it is vital.

Copper is found in all body tissues. During growth, the largest concentrations occur in the developing tissues.

It is also one of the most important blood antioxidants and prevents the rancidity of polyunsaturated fatty acids. It is a factor in maintaining healthy cell membranes.

If copper is absent in the cell then this can also cause anemia of a different kind in which the red blood cells are reduced in both size and number, with a lower hemoglobin content.

Hemoglobin, the oxygen carrier of the blood is manufactured from iron stored in the liver. While lack of iron is the basic cause of anemia, this deficiency can be caused by lack of copper because copper is the enzyme catalyst in the production and conversion of iron into hemoglobin in the liver. Therefore, taking iron supplements to overcome the anemia in this case is useless unless copper is present in sufficient quantity.

Another important function of copper is in the building of certain proteins and in particular keratin, the protein for fingernails and hair.

Lack of copper alters the physical structure of keratin, causing it to become brittle.

Copper is essential for many enzymes including enzymes that help produce hormones. The best sources of copper are organ meat and seafood.

Average Western diets provide 1.2mg of copper per day for males and 0.9mg for females. The official recommended intake is 1.5 to 3.0mg per day. So many people are likely to be deficient, though copper deficiency is difficult to measure.

The use of copper supplements in the colloidal form should always be used wherever possible, otherwise 0.5 to 3.0mg in the sulphate form, to bring copper intake up to the recommended level. Daily intake of 30mg show no toxicity.

According to Mr. Peter Bennett, a lecturer and specialist consultant in organic farming and agricultural ecology from Adelaide, South Australia, if garden soil is deficient in copper, sweet corn stems will have pale yellow leaves at the apex, tattered edges to the lower leaves, and shortening of the stems between the nodes or knots giving a generally stunted appearance. Orange, mandarin, grapefruit or lemon tree will have die-back, a condition in which the new shoots die back and smaller twiggy growth develops in a somewhat bunched effect lower down the branches; fruit that develops will likely show brown mottling of the skin which frequently cracks open.

Onions will feel like a rubber ball, and the thin flesh will have a creamy yellow color instead of the crisp pearly whiteness of a healthy onion.

Fluorine

In its active form, fluoride, is present in soil, water, plants and all animal tissue.

Minute amounts are found in nearly every human tissue, especially in the skeleton for the formation of strong, hard bones and for teeth which can resist decay.

Deficiencies, which are geographical, demand more dental work, and probably too brittle bones in the elderly, resulting in fractured hips and much disability.

Gallium

Reports suggest gallium may reduce brain cancers.

Germanium

This trace mineral is highly efficient electrical initiator; aids in oxygen utilization; enhances immune system function.

Gold

Gold has been shown to reduce active joint inflammation.

Indium

Short-term benefits as reported by many indium users include increased energy, reduced need for sleep, and an enhanced sense of well being - the "indium high."

Long-term benefits include a gradual correction of many chronic illnesses. This includes, but is not limited to, improved blood pressure, healthier body weight and a reversal of visible signs of aging. *Iodine* Is a trace mineral, most of which is converted into iodide in the body. It aids in the development and functioning of the thyroid gland and is an integral part of the thyroxine, a principal hormone produced by the thyroid gland.

Iodine plays an important role in regulating the body's production of energy, promotes growth and development and stimulates the rate of metabolism, helping the body burn excess fat.

Mentality, speech and the condition of hair, nails, skin and teeth are dependent upon a well functioning thyroid gland.

Iodine is required to make thyroid hormones, which in turn control all energy in the body.

Best source of iodine are edible seaweed and seafood. Even breathing sea air provides iodine.

Deficiency is uncommon now because of iodized salt. Our average daily iodine intake is now 250mcg for males and 170mcg for females, well above the RDA of 150mcg.

Supplements of 50-200mcg of iodine in the potassium iodide form is used for some athletes. Iodine is not very toxic up to 2000mcg daily, but will exacerbate acne, this is why it is preferred wherever possible to use the colloidal form of iodine. No acne exacerbation have been noticed or reported with this form.

Iron

Is a mineral concentrate in the blood, which is present in every living cell. It is the mineral that is found in the largest amounts in the blood.

Iron is necessary for the carrying and exchange of oxygen in the blood, and for many systems involving oxidation and its converse, reduction.

It is involved in respiration by being the main carrier vehicle for getting oxygen to all the cells in the body. It is essential to the oxidation of fatty acids.

The main function of iron is in the formulation of hemoglobin, the oxygen-carrying red pigment in the blood.

Iron is widely available in food, with heme iron from meat being the most bio-available. Heme is an iron-containing non-protein portion of the hemoglobin molecule wherein the iron is in the ferrous (Fe^{2+}) state. Despite all the iron pills doled out in this country, and iron fortification of food, many people are deficient. Iron supplements should not be taken except as part of a multi-mineral. Even 50mg of iron by itself can be toxic. It is also difficult for the body to get rid of and it is a potent source of bacterial growth.

It causes increased oxidation (free radical damage). 10-25mg of iron can be used. Apart from colloidal iron there are several forms of iron such ferrous fumarate, ferrous gluconate or iron picolinate form. Most researchers warn against supplementation except with the colloidal multi-mineral. Inorganic iron supplements as mentioned earlier are only absorbed at the rate of 10-12% by the body.

Lanthanum

May reduce chronic fatigue diseases.

Manganese

Manganese is required by all living organisms. It takes part in a number of enzymatic reactions. Deficiency in animals and birds affects bone, reproduction and brain function, with abnormalities of bony growth, stillbirths, early deaths and sterility of the mother, and convulsions.

Manganese plays an important role, as an antioxidant, in the prevention of free radicals as in oxidation. It has a role to play a part in the degenerative process called aging.

It also plays a role in activating numerous enzymes that are necessary for utilization of choline, biotin, thiamine and vitamin C complex.

It is a catalyst in the synthesis of fatty acids, cholesterol and mucopolysaccharides.

Manganese is needed for proper formation of bone and is essential for normal glucose metabolism.

It also forms part of an internal antioxidant, superoxide dismutase (SOD).

The best food source for manganese is organic whole grains and black tea. Average intake in Western diet is

2.7mg per day for men and 2.2mg per day for women. The amount of manganese required for optimum health is unknown. The RDA handbook recommends a provisional intake of 25mg per day.

Supplementation of 2-5mg of manganese can be used per day in the gluconate form if colloidal form is not readily available. Manganese is one of the least toxic minerals.

Molybdenum

It is found in practically all plant and animal tissues, but very scarce in the earth itself.

Molybdenum is involved in the final production stage of urine and helps promote normal cell function.

Molybdenum forms part of three essential enzymes.

Whole grains and legumes are the best sources of molybdenum but amounts vary widely in these foods, depending on the molybdenum content of the soil in which they are grown. The amount of molybdenum required for optimal health is unknown. Provisional RDA recommendation is 50-250mcg per day. 40-150mcg in the sodium molybdate form can be used per day, as part of a complete mineral supplement, when colloidal form is not available.

Molybdenum is not toxic up to 9mg per day. Above that it causes a gout-like condition.

Nickel

Nickel is an essential trace mineral found in the body. Human and animal tests show that nickel may be a factor in hormone, lipid and membrane metabolism as well as cell membrane integrity.

Significant amounts are found in DNA and RNA. Nickel may act as a stabilizer of these nucleic acids.

Selenium

Selenium is an essential mineral found in minute amounts in the body. It is one of the essential body substances used in a preventive manner for many diseases, including cancer, heart disease, muscular dystrophy, arteriosclerosis, stroke, cirrhosis, cataracts, arthritis and emphysema.

Selenium appears to preserve elasticity of tissue that becomes less elastic with aging. All diseases that are associated with aging are affected by the workings of selenium. Selenium functions either alone or with enzymes. Selenium forms part of key enzymes in the body for its work as a natural antioxidant that protects against free radicals.

Selenium is widespread in food, but deficient in the soil of many countries, especially New Zealand, so it is also deficient in the livestock and produce grown on those soils.

Average daily intake in the U.S. is about 108mcg. Because of our increased needs for antioxidants this amount is likely to be insufficient.

200-400mcg per day of selenium in the L-selenium-methionine form is used for therapeutic purposes. For prevention measures we prefer and recommend colloidal mineral supplementation that contains selenium. Selenium can be very toxic in excess of 800mcg per day, especially in the sodium selenite form. In some countries, such as Australia, selenium is not available in health stores or pharmacies. It can be obtained only through medical prescription.

Silica

Silica increases collagen in growing bones by 100%.

Silicon

Silicon is present in the tissues of skin, fingernails, bones, lungs, trachea, lymph nodes, tendons and aorta. The lungs have highest concentration because of their exposure to the air.

Silver

Silver kills over 650 disease causing organisms; systemic disinfectant and immune support. It subdues inflammation and promotes healing as well as acting as an anti-bacterial, anti-viral and anti-fungal.

Sodium

Is an essential mineral that is found in every cell in the body, predominantly in the extracellular fluids, the vascular fluids within the blood vessels, arteries, veins and capillaries, and the intestinal fluids surrounding the cells. It functions with potassium to equalize the acid-alkali factor in the blood.

Along with potassium, it helps regulate fluid balance within the body and the distribution of fluids on either side of the cell walls. Sodium, potassium and chloride are three main electrolytes. They perform multiple essential functions, without which life would end in an instant.

Sodium is the main cation (positively charged electrolyte) outside cells.

So much sodium is added to our food that the average Western diet consumes more than 5 grams per day, 10 times the recommended amount for good health. Avoid taking salt pills and extra salt. Excessive sodium raises blood pressure and has pathological effects.

In our over salted diet, a low sodium diet is a basic principle of good health. Try cooking without salt, and learn to enjoy the flavor of real food. Avoid adding salt to the meal before having tasted it.

Strontium

As essential trace element, strontium can replace calcium in many organisms including man.

Sulfur

Sulfur is an important mineral used in several amino acids involved in functions of hemoglobin, insulin hormone, adrenal hormones, enzymes and antibodies.

Tin

Animal studies show deficiencies in tin cause poor growth and poor feeding, hearing loss and male pattern baldness. Tin may have cancer prevention properties.

Vanadium

Vanadium aids in glucose (blood sugar) oxidation and transport and enhances insulin effectiveness (aids with blood sugar problems).

Vanadium decreases cholesterol production, increases effectiveness of heart muscle contraction and has anti-cancer properties.

Vanadium is an essential mineral involved in fat metabolism and is also found to protect the body against heart disease and cancer. Recently, the

University of Vancouver School of Medicine in British Columbia, conducted a study on insulin dependant diabetics. They found that in larger doses, vanadium can actually be used in place of insulin and helps to rebuild pancreatic tissue damaged through chromium and vanadium deficiency.

Zinc

Zinc is an essential trace mineral occurring in the body in larger amounts than any other trace element except iron. It is present in all tissues.

Zinc appears to be necessary for the building of protein, which makes up most of the solid matter of the cells. It is a constituent of: the enzyme which releases carbon dioxide from bicarbonate in the blood; the one which begins the oxidation of alcohol; other natural substances; and the splitting of portions of proteins.

Zinc is known for its ability to fight disease and to protect the immune system.

Zinc is involved in the Krebs cycle of energy production (Krebs cycle named after biochemist H.A. Krebs - 1900-1981 - a cyclic series of biochemical reactions, usually in the mitochondria, that represents the final common pathway in all aerobic organisms for the oxidation of amino acids, fats, and carbohydrates, and also converts the citric acid, etc. from food into carbon dioxide and ATP energy). More recently, blindness in the elderly has been found to be arrested by zinc. The visual part of the eye contains up to 4 percent zinc. It occurs in high amounts in the eyes of all species including fish.

Almost all of the zinc is inside the cells, where it is more abundant than any other trace element. Human and animal sperm contain large amounts of zinc, up to 0.2 percent. It is also credited with increasing male sex drive and potency because of its ability to regulate testosterone in the prostate. Zinc forms part of many essential enzymes, that catalyze (speed up) body functions, especially cell growth, skin repair, elasticity, immunity, testosterone production, sperm formation and sexuality.

It is vital for all metabolic processes including DNA synthesis, function and growth of the reproductive organs, wound healing, carbohydrate metabolism and protection against birth defects.

The World Health Organization ranks the United States as the highest in incidence of birth defects of 33 nations surveyed. In America, there is one human baby born with a birth defect for every 5,000 births. Compare this to the animal husbandry industry which has one birth defect for every 500,000 births! Steers raised for slaughter are fed a daily diet containing 40 to 50 minerals, but infant formula fed to human babies does not contain more than 12 minerals.

A zinc deficiency is related to diseases such as cystic fibrosis, can retard growth, cause skin lesions, brittle hair and nails.

Body stores of zinc are small and have to be replaced constantly by zinc from daily nutrition.

Best sources of zinc are meat, eggs, nuts and seafood.

Studies of zinc intake in average diets report only 8.5mg per day, well below the male RDA of 15mg. So deficiency is rampant.

Zinc supplements of 15-50mg in the picolinate form is used when colloidal form is not available. Toxicity of zinc is low, up to 500mg per day. Research has shown that zinc should not be taken except as part of a multi-mineral supplement.

Excess zinc disrupts copper metabolism, which disrupts iron metabolism causing a chain reaction with other minerals. Prolonged excess of single minerals leads to serious health problems.

Other Minerals

Cobalt forms an essential part of vitamin B12.

Nickel and arsenic (trace levels of course) are essential for normal growth in animals. This is important for many bio-electrical functions. It aids immune system activity, enhances hair growth and improves reflexes.

In todays day and age of sophisticated marketing and health obsession one must be careful to avoid scams. Not all mineral supplements are what they claim to be. Especially when it comes to new generations such as colloidal mineral solutions. Make sure you know what you are buying and, if still in doubt, look up references and do not hesitate to ask questions. In this way both money and health will be saved.

Currently no known function in the human body: Barium, Bismuth, Bromine, Cadmium, Cerium, Iridium, Niobium, Osmium, Palladium, Platinum, Rhodium, Rubidium, Tellurium, Titanium, Tungsten, Uranium, or Zirconium.

Minerals as Electrolytes

The source of electrolytes is minerals in our rocks, sand and soils. These have to be converted by plants to enable the body to produce electrolytes.

Metal atoms in minerals are the centers of electro-charge in large molecules that form cells and living tissues.

Metal elements coordinate and direct the flow of electrons, reactions between atoms, strength of membranes, and action of enzymes in biological life.

An ion is an atom that gains or loses one or more electrons. Since such an atom then has an excess or shortage of electrons in outer orbits circling around the nucleus, an ion has electric charge. This gives ions the essential energy needed to power chemical reactions.

Some elements - mostly metals - easily release electrons to have positive charge: a cation (+). Others - mostly minerals - capture extra electrons to acquire negative charge: an anion (-).

For example, sodium (Na), one of the lightest metals, easily gives up the single, unpaired electron in its outer-most orbital to become a cation (Na). But the positive charge is so strong it rapidly reacts and bonds with other atoms. Tossed in water, a pure pellet reacts with such quick vigor it explodes with a loud, violent pop! So, we seldom encounter sodium as pure metal, only as its mineral salts.

Similarly, most metals react with oxygen, hydrogen, nitrogen, sulfur, chlorine, etcetera, to become minerals. These crystal chemicals become earths bedrock, boulders, stone, soil, sand, silt, salt, clay, dirt, and dust.

Natural Versus Metallic

Whereas metallic minerals maybe toxic, colloidal minerals are nontoxic, due to their electrical charge and plant origin. A good example is iodine which is harmless and beneficial whereas two or three grains of free iodine will kill you. The same is true for lead, arsenic, aluminum, and other minerals considered toxic.

Salts of the Earth

Nature and biology are too tender for the extreme energy concentrated in mineral salts, so cellular chemistry employs gentler ways to exchange electrons and empower reactions.

In the simple chemistry of inorganic minerals, an electrolyte is an ionic substance which dissolves in water. These ions-in-solution are valuable for their effects on waters electrical properties. Most often, they increase waters ability to pass an electric current, or store electric charge.

Simple electrolytes can be three types:

acid (+)

base (-) or alkali

salt (+) or neutral

These three classes of ionic chemicals are interrelated by a Chemical Cross. In this most fundamental chemical reaction, acid and base unite to form salt and water. Acid and base are polar, with opposite ionic charge, but salt - with both cations and anions - is neutral.

The Chemical Cross
salt y (H+) acid x w   Alkaline (OH-) z water
a common example: H+CI+ Na+OH-x Na+CI+ H2O   hydrogen sodium sodium water chloride hydroxide chloride
NOTE: hydrogen chloride is hydrochloric acid without water

Acid-base balance (or pH) - the most critical chemical characteristic -is measured as parts per million or H+ ions, and is rated on a 0 - to - 14 logarithmic scale in which 7.00 is neutral. Salt is chemical fire. Its corrosive appetite is fed - not by wood or coal - but by metals, whose electrons fuel chemical reactions.

To render this concept into sensation, take the taste test. After sodium chloride is refined out of sea salt, beige crystals remain. Refiners discard this residue as impurities, but natural food stores sell it as nigari to curdle soymilk into tofu. Mostly it is magnesium and calcium, but it also contains every minor and trace element found in seawater, minus the sodium.

Touch a crystal of this trace element salt to the tongue, and a sharp bite of hot, burning sensation will be felt. This fire is its power to cause chemical reactions - the exchange of electrons by metal elements. Every enzyme requires an electrolyte as its key component. Without this electric spark, there can be no taste, or smell, or sight. No sensation, or motion, or light. And no life.

Even slight alterations in concentrations of ionic chemicals in our body fluids will disturb vital cell functions. For example, low potassium ions cause general muscle paralysis, while high levels create weak, irregular heartbeats. Therefore, our body has evolved with multiple methods to maintain stable, constant levels of electrolytes in blood, lymph, and all other body fluids.

Electrolytes Source of Balance Critical to Good Health

Like spark plugs in a car, electrolytes supply the spark to trigger a myriad of reactions in cells. They deliver electrons where needed for reactions, and store charges between reactions (scientists estimate that ten thousand chemical reactions take place every minute of the day!).

Electrolytes sustain the most critical chemical balance in the body: pH - the acid-base balance- is a delicate chemical condition that determines how available electrons are for these reactions.

Too much positive charge (cations) from acids (+) creates an inability to circulate electrons. Excess negative charge (anions) of an alkaline state (-) will overcharge a cell or organism.

Life is a constant changing experience that survives by balance from reaction to reaction. Most biological processes need neutral - slightly alkaline - pH to assure a steady supply of electrons.

Our blood remains very close to 7.45 pH, a shift of 1 point can cause death. Electrolytes not only help restore neutral pH balance, they also act as buffers that resist any change in pH.

The neutral factor ensures that when food ingested is too acidic, the body can prevent a change in pH. A healthy body with electrolytes will temporarily neutralize these extremes.

Like earths polluted air, blood and lymph have become too acid - not occasionally, but chronically and critically. Like trees dying on high mountaintops from acid rain, intestinal micro-flora wilt and weaken if the pH of their environment changes.

When the pH of cell fluid becomes too acid, proteins change their shape, and many enzymes no longer function.

Most modern illness is due to disturbed pH. Infections, yeasts, parasites, and worms all thrive in an acid pH. Cancer, heart disease and arthritis are but a few of the diseases resulting from the inability to sustain a stable, neutral pH, and cell membrane integrity.

Osteoporosis is rampant in the United States, the wealthiest nation on the earth. Chronic excess acids force the body to use calcium stored in teeth and bones to neutralize acids.

Poor, depleted soil cannot supply minerals needed for electrolytes, while refining and processing remove even more minerals, so the electromagnetic charge cannot be generated. No matter how much we supplement, calcium cannot adhere to bone matrix without this electromagnetic force.

A cell's most critical function is to maintain the integrity of the cell membrane - the inner-outer pressure balance at a cell wall to separate cell from non-cell. This double layer of lipids of the cell membrane is in constant motion, fed by electrolytes. A strong membrane is a cells first line of defense - the frontline of the immune system. Without electrolytes, this barrier cannot be sustained, weakens, and a virus or bacteria can invade the cell.

Trace element crystalloid electrolytes are the key catalysts in thousands of enzymes needed by cells to make amino acids, proteins, and other organic molecules.

When electrolytes form, they generate more electro-chemical activity, attract more minerals, and capture more charge.

Electro charge control is the key to enzymes that allow biochemical reactions to occur rapidly, selectively and precisely. For example, zinc is used in over 20 enzyme systems.

The pancreas for example, produces enzymes and acids to break down food in digestion.

Drinking electrolytes 30 minutes before a meal moistens and recharges soft tissues lining the digestive tract. When food is ingested membranes and micro-organisms are ready to digest and absorb food.

Furthermore, electrolytes supply the pancreas new ions to make more digestive enzymes and hydrochloric acid.

Electrolytes are critical to nerves - both individually and collective coordination of the entire nervous system. Nerve impulses are transmitted as an exchange of sodium and potassium ions at the nerve membrane and through the nerve synapse centers. Nerve membrane is encased in long tendrils of protein with a calcium ion attached at the end of each strand. Without this impulse of ion charge, there can be no taste, smell, sight, sensation or awareness.

Hormones, vitamins and enzymes which activate, regulate and synchronize nerve action all require a mineral ion as key element in their reactive structure, and for their synthesis. For one, cobalt is needed by the pineal gland to make melatonin, the hormone regulating neurological function determining the level of sleep or wakefulness.

These are a few examples of the many intricate and essential role of these mineral ions in blood chemistry, cell biology, human physiology, brain psychology and global ecology.

Electrolytes are the key to unlock energy flow in a cell. This energy flow makes life happen.

Chapter 4
Cell Chemistry

A book on minerals would be incomplete without description of the complex chemistry of minerals and electrolytes. This is fascinating to read and more so to comprehend one of our creators amazing life-sustaining chemistries. Although this subject has become an advanced science, for a separate book, the author has attempted to present a simplified over view.

The shocking truth is this amazing chemistry is clearly one which is meant to maintain vibrant health when the electrolytes maintain an alkaline pH. When we ignore this fundamental principal with unnatural factors in our lifestyle, poor nutrition, exposure to chemicals and stress, this alkaline balance is altered due to a drain on the critical electrolytes responsible for maintaining the alkaline balance. The altered state, which is a shift to an acid pH is ill health, disease and premature death.

It is unforgivable that this simple principal is ignored by the medical establishment focussed on the treatment of illness and disease with medications and drugs that are in conflict with this natural chemistry. The use of medications and drugs worsen the imbalance to perpetuate the symptoms, suffering and hasten deaths.

To simplify this explanation certain key words need to be understood. Wherever possible this is included in the text and can also be found in the glossary.

To begin with:

1. When healthy, the pH of blood is 7.4, the pH of spinal fluid is 7.4, and the pH of saliva is 7.4. Thus, the pH of the saliva parallels the extracellular fluid. Calcium (mono) orthophosphate is a major component of these chemical buffer body fluids that tries to maintain the pH at 7.4.

2. This pH is critical in promoting normal DNA synthesis, cell growth, cell function, and cell repair. As the level of the chemical buffer drops in the serums, so too does the ability to maintain this critical pH. The calcium ion level therefore has a direct reflection on the pH. This can be measured by a simple three second, two cent, pH test of the saliva that provides an immediate indication of the state of the calcium ion level, and thus indirectly the state of our health (see appendix for explanation of pH saliva test).

3. Hundreds of scientific publications have been written describing the cell membrane ion channels or pores that allow entry of nutrients into the cell. Because of size, each channel is restrictive to specific ions. For example, a channel just big enough for sodium to enter would readily deny entry to the larger calcium ion and the much larger

potassium ion. These selective ion channels can be used to allow ions within the cell to exit, as the ions entering the cell are usually attached to large numbers of nutrient radicals and therefore require much larger channels. These large nutrient channels contain a rosette of five proteins each of which are bound in seven oxygen locations by the king of the bioelements, calcium. This causes the protein to bunch up, creating a plug that will shut off entry through the channel. As the nutrients within the cell undergo chemical reactions liberating their radical components that are to be used for cell growth and DNA synthesis, the attached calcium and other cations are also liberated.

This production of cations inside of the cell drops the pH from 7.4 to about 6.6 thereby giving the intracellular fluids a positive charge.

The pH of the fluids inside the cell drops from alkaline negative pH of 7.4 when the channels are open, so as to lower the acidic positive pH of the fluids to 6.6 after the channels close and the nutrients have been chemically altered and consumed by the cell.

This change in pH creates the potential difference (voltage) between the inside cellular fluids and the outside fluids, resulting in the channels opening again. This process is repeated indefinitely like a cell breathing process. When discharged into the cell, this electrical potential activates all the biological processes that are responsible for cell function and nerve stimulus.

However, if the pH of the extracellular fluids falls to a level lower than 7.4, say to a pH 0f 6.5 due to chronic calcium deficiency, then the intracellular fluids must drop lower, to about 6.3 to produce the same electrical voltage difference. This causes the nutrient glucose to stop producing the A, C, G and T radicals required for normal DNA synthesis, and instead to produce lactic acid, which drops the pH even further. The result is a weakening of the cell function. If the extracellular pH drops even further, the intracellular pH drops correspondingly, and may result in the production of toxic enzymes as well as cellular breakdown.

These alterations manifest as disease, the aging process, and the production of cell mutations.

The impact of this alteration:

The illustration above emphasizes that pH alkaline balance maintains good health and that degenerative disease thrives in acidic body fluids. There are factors that can explain some of the many reasons for this phenomenon:

1. As is described in more detail in Chapter 6, cancer, bacteria, and virus cannot survive in oxygen. One important biochemical reaction with alkaline fluids is a capacity to absorb oxygen and other gasses. For example, some alkaline fluids have many times more capacity to absorb oxygen than acidic fluids. Thus, the oxygen-rich, alkaline body fluids are more capable of killing a virus than oxygen poor, acidic body fluids.

2. Therefore biological functions prefer alkaline fluids because alkalines are hydroxides which are composed of oxygen and hydrogen.

3. The surface membrane of each cell is composed of a bi-layer of phospholipids which could be compared

to an air mattress composed of upper and lower layers fused together by a cholesterol substance.

The surface of the phospholipid layers contains significant oxygen generating a hydrophilic state, or, in other words, water and fluids attract to it.

This layer of oxygen is very negatively charged, thereby allowing the surface to capture positive cancer causing chemicals, most of which are made up of derivatives of the electron-starved benzene. These positively charged carcinogens stick to the negatively charged surface, and, like flies to flypaper, are eliminated from any activity. The cell surface can hold a lifetime of these carcinogens, within reasonable limits, but unlike the flypaper that holds the flies until they die, the cell only holds the carcinogens until the cell dies and disintegrates. Once liberated, the carcinogen can get inside the ruptured cell, where it induces cell mutation.

The oxygen rich, negatively charged cell surface also attracts the positively charged minerals, such as calcium and magnesium, which then attract negatively charged nutrients in preparation for entry into the cell. This initiates a biological exchange that is life itself as explained as follows:

These nutrients enter the cell through a nutrient channel which is kept closed by a rosette of coiled proteins, like a coiled snake plugging a hole, bound together by calcium.

When the rosette snake uncoils, it makes an opening which allows the mineral stacked nutrients to enter the cell. The rosette of proteins coils or stretches as required because the changing chemical charges.

The difference between the slightly acidic pH of the fluid inside the cell, which continues to drop as the nutrients inside are consumed in biochemical reactions, and the constantly high pH of 7.4 of the fluids outside the cell, generates an electrical potential difference (an electrical voltage).

When the charge becomes large enough, it causes the positively charged end of the rosette snake to coil to stretch towards the negatively charged external fluids, thereby opening the cell and allowing the higher pH nutrients to flow through the nutrient channel into the cell.

These high pH fluids entering the cell in turn raise the pH inside the cell, thereby lowering the electrical charge, allowing the rosette snake to recoil and plug the channel.

Thus the cell has been opened and closed electrically. Therefore, electro-physiology is a reality. One can easily imagine an external electrical charge superimposing its negative voltage on the cell, causing it to remain open. The result would be biological havoc.

When the main nutrient, which is the sugar glucose, enters the cell, it begins to undergo immediate changes that are dependent on the pH or degree of acidity inside the cell. For example, if the inner cell fluids are at a pH of 6.0 or lower, the acid causes the six carbon glucose to split in half, forming two lactic acid molecules (each containing three carbons), which thereby drops the pH even further. This acid results in cell surface disintegration which liberates the carcinogens and toxins for entry into the ruptured cell. If, on the other hand, the fluids inside the cell are at the more alkaline pH of 6.5 or higher, only one or two of the carbons are removed from the six carbon glucose. This can allow the four nucleotides containing 4 and 5 carbons, which are the basic building blocks of DNA, to be formed. Thus, in an acidic environment, the DNA which is Mother Nature's blueprint for the body, cannot be formed. This is probably the main reason why acidosis results in degenerative diseases, and why raising the body fluid's pH can result in curing the disease.

1. The production of cations inside of the cell drops the pH from 7.4 to about 6.6, thereby giving the intracellular fluids a positive charge. (A solution with a pH of less than 7.0 is positive and a solution with a pH greater than 7.0 is negative. Thus, the extracellular fluids with a pH of 7.4 are negative.)

2. What is very important to understand is with the extracellular fluid negative and the intracellular fluid positive, the potential of electrocharge or voltage is about 17 millivolts. This level is what exerts a pull at each end of the charged rosette of proteins blocking the channel, causing it to stretch and thereby to open up the channel.

Impact on Aging

Acidosis prevents the formation of nucleotides, which are the building blocks of DNA, which is the blueprint for human growth, thereby slowing down growth and body repair, which are two of the basic traits of aging. This is probably why people who are very sick with disease look very old, and when health returns, they regain some youth. What this means to the layperson is that there really may be a fountain of youth, and it would be in the form of alkaline body fluids.

Summary of pH:

3. Electrolytes maintain pH.

4. pH creates electrical charge essential to the delivery and transport of nutrients into the cell.

5. The alkaline pH and the negative charge of the cell membrane attract carcinogens. When pH becomes acid, DNA function is altered and disease, aging and cancer follow.

Chapter 5
The Synergistic Impact of Water

Water is a component of the trilogy - oxygen, minerals and water - of the essential elements indispensable to life.

Water provides the fluids in the many systems of the body acting as the transport system for minerals, oxygen and nutrients to the cells and as the fluid essential to remove toxins out of the body.

What is not understood is that these fluids need to be maintained at a level for efficient functioning of body systems and the transport of the essential minerals.

Water is a tasteless, odorless, colorless liquid, used as the standard of specific gravity as well as specific heat. It is present in all organic tissues in many other substances, and is the most universal of solvents.

Drinking Water - Mineral Content of Water

A 1992 study published in a European Journal of Heart Disease revealed a relationship to minerals in the water of 76 Swedish communities. Cities with the highest mineral content had the lowest incidence of heart disease.

The same scientists studied enzymes that keep Eskimo arteries clean. Eskimos eat a high fat diet, yet still maintain excellent health, because they eat a natural, highly mineralized diet, their bodies produce the necessary enzymes.

It will probably be surprising to read that water is not only essential for survival, the body requires a daily intake adequate to support every function and cellular activity to maintain a healthy body. Inadequate daily water intake is a determining factor in the development of illness and disease.

When illness and disease has appeared water should become an important priority. Inadequate water may delay healing even when other measures are correctly implemented. Like the blood, if not maintained at a certain volume or if it becomes poisoned with toxic waste it, will lead to serious disease and subsequent death.

It is true to say that water is a determining factor of health and disease. This chapter explains why. The author has demonstrated in workshops that the information presented here explains an important factor contributing to altered chemistry and chronic stress in the development of cancer as well as the impact when water intake is used to support oncological treatment.

The distribution and transport of water is a complex chemistry regulating all functions throughout the body. Water is a transporter of vital nutrients to every cell and system. Water is a solvent in the chemistry assimilating minerals in which they become electrolytes needed to activate many biochemical checks and balances such as pH, metabolic and hormonal systems.

Through a system of osmotic transfer, water transports minerals across membranes and maintains a balance such as sodium chloride extracellular and potassium and magnesium intracellular.

The author reports that there is increasing evidence that cancer patients who have overcome the disease have focussed on maximizing the potential of the healing power of the trilogy described here!

Having made the above statements, some knowledge about the chemistry and function of water is necessary to comprehend the importance of water in both the development of illness and disease (as in dehydration) and as the healer.

Real life research and experience indicates that dehydration due to inadequate water intake is a major factor in the development of many types of cancer. Typically this is a process over a number of years during which time many different kinds of symptoms appear particularly those that are labeled of unknown etiology.

Generally, perception is limited to the body as a muscular-skeletal system making up the solid structure and appearance, and water is necessary and is passed out in the form of urine.

In fact 75% of the muscles, 83% of the kidneys, 22% of the bones and 72% of blood is water. Even the brain is as high as 85% water (although the brain is only 1/50th of the weight of the body it receives 18-20 % of blood circulation). In total, weight water is as much as 60% 70% of body weight.

Water makes everything happen in the body. Water is distributed throughout the body in every cell, in the muscle tissues, in the bones and even the teeth. Water is responsible for transport of essential nutrients, temperature control, blood pressure, detoxification, electrolyte and pH balance. Essential functions that maintain life such as the pumping of the heart; every movement of the body is dependent on the presence and regulation of water. Water regulates the function of the kidneys essential to fluid balance and detoxification of wastes.

The great bulk of living matter is just plain water, yet historically, the subject of water and electrolyte balance is a newcomer to the art and science of biological medicine. This is not to imply, of course, that our grandparents did not know enough to take a drink of water to quench their thirst. Indeed they did - but often to their detriment! Drinking plain water in response to excessive sweating for example, results in heat cramps unless salt is also taken. Today this is common knowledge - sweat contains salt as well as water - but years ago this relationship was not understood.

It was just about fifty years ago that patients in hospital began to receive the benefits of both salt and water in the treatment and prophylaxis of dehydration. Eventually the shortcomings of plain salt and water were revealed and the complexities of body fluid disturbances brought to light. Protracted diarrhea, for example, can be fatal despite the replacement of salt and water unless the doctor also administers potassium and bicarbonate. Conversely, the administration of potassium to a patient with acute renal disease can cause immediate death. In this chapter, we go beyond simply understanding the electrolyte chemistry of the body and the impact of water and explain how inadequate water leads to levels of dehydration with serious consequences.

The subject of body fluids - that is, water and electrolytes - is of life and death importance and becomes especially important in the treatment of dehydration in all of its many forms.

Our approach will be as follows: First, to understand the basic facts of body water, body ions, and body pH in health and disease and then to apply this knowledge to the basic treatment of specific diseases.

Balance and Osmosis

There is a miraculous structure in which the body is able to maintain - or balance - fluid compartments at their respective volumes.

The boundary between the intracellular (in the cells) and intercellular (outside cells) compartments is the sum total of all the cellular membranes. Regulating compartmental water balance is a function of the cellular membrane which is, among a myriad other things, semipermeable; that is, it easily permits the free movement of water molecules, but partially or completely prevents the passage of other particles.

When such a membrane separates two aqueous solutions with different densities, the principal flow of water across the membrane will be in the direction of the solution with the greater density (density or osmotic density, means the proportion of particles - ions and molecules -to volume). This will continue until the two solutions are of the same density, at which time the rate of flow will be the same in both directions.

Osmosis

The flow of water across a semi-permeable membrane as a consequence of a difference in density is called osmosis, and the rule is, as just stated, that the principal flow will be from the less dense to the more dense. There is one way to remember this and that is: the least dense solution has the most water.

In health, the concentration of the intracellular compartments is such that at osmotic equilibrium the water distribution is 15 percent intracellular and 40 percent extracellular. When these concentrations are disturbed, problems can be expected.

Plasma Compartment

Plasma is 90% water. Plasma also contains protein, dissolved salts and minerals including sodium, calcium, magnesium and potassium as well as antibodies.

Shifting our attention, note that the intercellular compartment membrane borders the plasma compartment as well as the intracellular compartment, thereby interacting as a second osmotic system - the capillary wall serving as the semi-permeable membrane.

Here water is forced out of the capillaries by the hydrostatic pressure of the blood and pulled into the capillaries by osmotic (or oncotic; pertaining to, caused by or marked by swelling; the osmotic pressure due to the presence of colloids in a solution; in the case of plasma - interstitial fluid interaction, it is the force that tends to counterbalance the capillary blood pressure) pull of plasma protein.

Essentially, the maintenance - and balance - of the water content of the plasma (5%) and intercellular (15%) compartments depends upon the blood pressure and plasma protein concentration. For example, in malnutrition, there is a drop in plasma protein with the result that excessive amounts of water are lost to the intercellular compartment, causing edema and swollen bellies. Conversely, in dehydration, the loss of water from the plasma causes a relative increase in protein concentration with the result that water, this time, is lost to the capillaries.

Water Intoxication

Let us now integrate this information about compartmental balance by considering an actual derangement. The drinking of large amounts of water over and above what the body needs can cause a serious condition called water intoxication. This is what happens; water taken into the body is absorbed into the blood - the plasma compartment - thus increasing blood volume and, thereby, blood pressure.

As a result of this increased pressure, water is forced through the capillary walls into the intercellular compartment. The intercellular compartment now becomes more dilute, meaning that water will leave it and pass into the now relatively more concentrated intracellular compartment. Thus, the underlying pathology of water intoxication is excessive cellular hydration. But of chief interest at this point is that an alteration in one compartment is reflected by alterations in the other two. One further example should crystallize this fact.

When a person drinks an excessive amount of salt water, the kidney is not able to prevent a build-up of salt in the intracellular compartment with the result that water will be withdrawn from the intracellular compartment into the intercellular and plasma compartments, in that order. This means, of course, that the blood pressure will increase (as a result of an increase of blood volume) and the output of urine will be increased. Indeed, for each quart of seawater the castaway drinks, he eliminates a quart and a half of urine, with the difference coming from the cells. Cause of death - dehydration - an alteration in one compartment causes alterations in the other two.

The above describes three osmotic compartments as follows:

1   Intracellular
2   Intercellular
3   Plasma

Although the above example explains the impact of excessive water intake, this section describes the impact of inadequate water which is little understood and affects most every person on this planet.

Impact of Dehydration on Cancer

An important explanation of the impact of water in the development of cancer and degenerative disease follows:

1. Inadequate water is a stress resulting in a hormone response that breaks down tissue to release cellular water. Therefore, inadequate water adds to the catabolic damage, weakening the body to become more vulnerable to the development of the disease.

On the opposite side, adequate water minimizes such breakdown and allows the body to respond to healing, especially when healing foods make available water and the essential nutrients especially minerals, to become ionized and converted to electrolytes.

2. High protein food, especially complete protein as in eggs, and food that supply minerals and enzymes (fresh vegetables and fruit) work to reverse this degenerative process. The challenge is to correctly determine the correct combination, quantity and frequency.

3. In the process of cellular breakdown (catabolic) there is release of toxic ashes. This release of toxins adds to the problem, as more water is needed to flush these toxins out of the body or transfer them to other systems to be broken down. The greater the level of toxic build-up the greater the acceleration of degenerative disease.

4. Other sections of this book explain how stress mechanisms trigger hormone response to convert glycogen reserves to energy to respond to the demands of stress. When these reserves are inadequate hormones break down cellular tissue to release resources in response to stress demands. This break down releases toxins adding to the additional demand for water which, if not adequate, increases the toxic load factor detrimental to healing.

5. The consequence of this break down of the osmotic membrane leads to an alteration of the intracellular and intercellular balance.

Another important fact is that this catabolic process appears to target weak sites. That explains how the numerous different kinds of cancers occur.

The author emphasizes that his opinion is that here lies the explanation of the change in chemistry leading to the development of malignancy. Further explanation follows:

As a result of the catabolic attack leading to a breakdown of the permeable osmotic membrane, the damaged cells allow the flow of intercellular (situated between the cells of any structure) fluid into the cells resulting in three serious changes intracellularly (situated or occurring within a cell or cells).

a. Increase of sodium causing imbalance with other electrolytes especially potassium.

b. The entry of virus leading to an attack on the DNA thereby the uncontrolled development affecting surrounding cells in the development of malignancy and tumors.

c. Alteration and derangement of the electromagnetic fields that generate energy.

From the above explanation the impact of dehydration leads to the following:

a. Inadequate daily intake of water leads to increased stress ranging from hormonal, to the elevated levels of toxins, inefficient detoxification and poor delivery of essential nutrients.

b. A catabolic breakdown of the protective membranes leading to cellular damage, altered homeostasis affecting the DNA and development of uncontrolled malignant cells.

c. Catabolic damage releases toxic ashes adding to the toxic load.

d. It is clear that effective therapy must reverse this process. This means rehydration, detoxification, a high nutrition diet supplying high easily digested complete protein (legumes, grains, cereals, eggs), and vegetable food rich in minerals (raw vegetables, fruit).

e. Many other approaches to treating cancer fail because the above rehydration and restoration of homeostasis is not achieved. On the other hand, cancer responds more successfully to oncology when rehydration and nutrients as described above are administered.

f. Clearly, the more damage due to dehydration the more the demand for nutrition. Factors preventing intake of high nutrition will compromise success. This is dramatically illustrated when advanced cancer patients are fed high protein nutrition food blends through tube feeding frequently throughout the day.

Water Movement and Transport

There is an amazing transport and regulating chemistry that shifts water to stress sites and changing circumstance to anabolic and metabolic functions.

In the internal system there is constant absorption of water and delivery to the blood system. Exogenous (produced outside the body) and endogenous (produced inside the body) toxins accumulate in the colon. This is especially problematical when water is inadequate.

The case is overwhelmingly in favor of:

a. Oncology Support Programs in collaboration with Oncologists

b. Integrated HealthCare - parenteral nutrition, detoxification, colon hydrotherapy, and stress management.

Water Substitutes

Thinking that tea, coffee, alcohol and manufactured beverages are substitutes for natural water needs of the body is an elementary mistake in advanced societies. It is true that these beverages contain water, but they also contain additives that include dehydrating agents. Studies demonstrate they result in water loss equal to that taken plus more water from the reserves of the body! Today, modern life-style makes people dependent on a variety of beverages. Children are not educated to drink water; they become dependent on sodas. This is a self-imposed restriction on the water needs of the body. It is also not generally possible to drink manufactured products in full replacement of the water needs of the body. At the same time, a cultivated preference for the taste of these sodas will automatically reduce the free urge to drink water when sodas are not available or the costs of 8-plus cans daily a consideration.

Distilled Water

Another problem in conflict with electrolyte balance is the perception that drinking distilled water is responding to our understanding of the importance of water supply to the body. It is disturbing that many who drink distilled water are health conscious and work to drink much more than others.

Distilled water is lifeless dead fluid without minerals which have been removed in the distillation process. The more distilled water consumed, the more leaching out of minerals from the mineral reserves. Leaching out of minerals is particularly severe for those living in a hot climate due to increased level of mineral lost in sweating. When clean well or natural spring water is not available at least one should do is to add crystalloid electrolyte solution (about 3 teaspoons to one gallon water).

Symptoms of Dehydration

Because most practitioners of medicine are unaware of the many biochemical roles of water, symptoms of dehydration are translated as indicators of unknown metabolic or disease conditions of the body. As a result, medical practitioners do not advise preventive measures; nor do they offer effective measures to hydrate the body so essential to healing.

Medications used to treat the symptoms add to the problem, and accelerate development of pathology. However, when used in conjunction with rehydration, balance occurs and medications are no longer needed.

Alimentary Balance

A special form of compartmental balance is the relationship between plasma water and alimentary secretions - the latter being derived from the former. According to J.L. Gamble, the total volume of alimentary secretions during twenty-four-hour period may reach the staggering volume of 8200 ml or 8.2 liters and, what is more, all but about 150ml is returned to the circulation for reabsorption in the intestine. No wonder, that protracted vomiting or diarrhea - without fluid replacement - can cause death in a matter of hours. About this, much more will be said for fluid derangements, in the wake of such alimentary losses and the treatment thereof.

Water Intake Versus Water Output

Living organisms vary tremendously in their water requirements. Whereas cactus can live for twenty-nine years on an amount of water equal to its own weight, it takes a human only a month to drink his/her weight in water. Regardless of the intake of quantity, the body normally balances the gain with an equivalent loss, or, explained another way, the body takes in an amount of water equal to that which it loses. The important objective is to maintain balance; the body is outstandingly successful in this regard. At twenty-four-hour intervals man's weight may vary less than one-half pound! The regulating mechanisms involved are discussed in the pages to follow.

In a typical day a person should gain as much as 3 liters. This includes:

- a) Water intake by mouth approximately, 1.5 liters a day.

- b) Water trapped in food makes up about half this amount (food accounts for a surprisingly high amount of water. For example - green vegetables about 95%, meat 55 -75%).

- c) Or derived from the oxidization of food. Oxidative water refers to water formed as a by-product in the body's oxidation of food. This amounts to about half of the preformed water in the food.

Roughly, the above three sources amount to an easy to remember ratio 4-2-1 (by mouth, food and oxidation). Thus the amount of food intake has a great bearing on the body's water needs for intake by mouth. Water by mouth is rapidly absorbed into the plasma compartment; in the absence of food. The process takes less than an hour.

It is clear that a person who skips breakfast, has two or three cups of coffee or tea, a skimpy lunch with tea or coffee and relies on the main meal at the end of the day, is not getting 3 liters water a day.

It is also appropriate to point out that the six meals per day are recommended and it relates to the contribution of water as a healer particularly in correcting or protection against dehydration. Furthermore, it also emphasizes that refined processed food lacks the natural food composition with the water content explained above.

Output

Now let us take a look at the body's water output. To balance the intake, the output runs close to 3 liters in a typical day. As one would guess, the kidneys carry the heaviest load (e.g. 1.7 liters). The other channels of excretion are not as apparent, but nonetheless vital. Under usual conditions, the body loses about 0.5 liter from the skin and 0.4 liter from the lungs. The remainder, 0.2 liter or so, is lost in the feces.

In contrast to fecal water and urine, the water loss via the lungs is in the form of vapor. Water lost through the skin is usually vapor, but can turn into water (sweat) when the body becomes overheated. The term *insensible perspiration* is used when referring to invisible sweat, or water vapor.

The Kidney and Water Balance

One of the functions of the kidney is to maintain water and electrolyte balance. For this reason special attention must be paid to this important system and to its relationship to other forces in the body. However, a shortfall in daily water intake results in severe stress and leads to many problems.

The Skin and Lungs

Whereas the healthy kidney always operates to maintain water balance, the same cannot be said of the skin. The loss of water through the skin serves not only to remove waste, but also to maintain body temperature. For example, in hot climates, while the kidney fights dehydration by putting out a low volume of urine, the skin fights the heat by allowing 10 to 12 liters of water to evaporate per day!

The sweat, or sudoriferous, glands lie deep in the true skin and their secretions - perspiration - are carried to the surface by corkscrew-like ducts. The work of these glands is governed by sympathetic nerves which, in turn, are under the direction of a hypothetical sweat center in the brain (perhaps in the hypothalamus). As the temperature of the blood rises, chiefly in response to the external temperature and/or muscular activity, the heat center is triggered to send impulses via sympathetic fibers to the glands. Sweat is thus formed and the body is cooled by evaporation. The sweat seen in many emotional conditions - the cold sweat of fear, for example - is easily explained by the emergency nature of the sympathetic system.

Perspiration, about 99 percent water, contains dissolved salts (chiefly NaCl - sodium chloride) and traces of urea. In abnormal conditions, however, bile pigments, albumin, sugar or even blood may appear in perspiration. The output on a typical day ranges around 0.5 liter.

The water lost by the lungs averages about 0.4 liters per day. Since this is a case of simple evaporation, the loss is constant and largely unaffected by other factors.

Water has Other Important Properties

Scientific research shows that water has many other properties besides being a solvent and a means of transport. It has an essential hydrolytic role in all aspects of body metabolism-water-dependent chemical reactions (hydrolysis).

At the cell membrane, the osmotic flow of water can generate hydroelectric energy (voltage gradient) that is stored in the energy pools in the form of ATP (adenosine triphosphate) - a compound of adenosine containing three phosphoric acid groups. This substance is present in all cells, but particularly in muscle cells. When this substance is split by enzyme action, energy is produced and used for elemental (cation) exchanges, particularly in neurotransmission.

ATP is a chemical source of energy in the body. The energy generated by water helps manufacture ATP.

Water also forms a particular pattern and shape that seems to be employed as the adhesive material in the bonding of the cell architecture.

Water Transport from the Brain

Biochemicals manufactured in the brain cells are transported to their destination in the nerve endings for use in the transmission of messages on waterways. There appears to be small waterways or micro-streams along the length of nerves that float materials along guidelines, called microtubules.

Impact on Proteins and Enzymes

Proteins and enzymes function more efficiently in solutions of lower viscosity (physical property of fluids that determines the internal resistance to shear forces); this is true of all the receptors in the cell membranes. In solutions of higher viscosity (in hydrated state) the proteins and enzymes become less efficient. It follows that water itself regulates all functions of the body, including the activity of all the solutes it carries around. It is clear that water - the solvent of the body, which regulates all functions, including the activity of the solutes it dissolves and circulates - should become a priority in future medical research.

Water and the Brain

Pathology that is seen to be associated with fear, anxiety, insecurity, persistent emotional and matrimonial problems - and depression are most often the result of water deficiency affecting the brain. The brain uses electrical energy that is generated by the water transport of the energy generating pumps. With dehydration, the level of the energy generation to the brain is decreased.

Many functions of the brain that depend on this type of energy become inefficient. This inadequacy of function is described as depression. This depressive state caused by dehydration can lead to chronic fatigue syndrome. This condition is a label for a number of advanced physiological problems that are seen to be associated with stress.

If the events are understood that take place in stress, we will also understand chronic fatigue syndrome. Many case studies demonstrate reversal of dehydration leads to disappearance of chronic fatigue and its metabolic complications. The following pages define the physiological events and the possible metabolic over-rides that can lead to the depletion of certain body reserves that may be the basic problem in chronic fatigue syndrome.

The Initial Silent Compensation Mechanisms Associated with Dehydration

When the body becomes dehydrated, the physiological processes are similar to the response coping with stress. Dehydration equals stress and, once established, there is an associated mobilization of resources from body stores. This process will absorb some water reserves of the body. Consequently, dehydration causes stress and stress will cause further dehydration.

Endorphins, Cortisone, Prolactin, and Vasopressin

A short explanation of these hormones is important as they impact the development of the disease. Keep in mind that stress has a cumulative damage determined by the duration of the stress response, the number of stress factors and the frequency. The response to stress is supposed to be short term. When stress is constant as in the development of dehydration and worse when cancer appears, the damage resulting from the cumulative constant demands of stress is the obstacle against healing. It follows that healing must work to remove stress (dehydration) and provide the body with maximum resources so as to minimize damage and maximize healing.

Hormonal glands and particularly hormones themselves need trace minerals to function. Continuing stress is another drain on the mineral reserve.

Endorphins

Endorphins prepare the body to endure hardship and injury until the assault has passed or healing has repaired the damage. They also raise the pain threshold.

Because of childbirth and monthly menstruation, women seem to access this hormone much more readily. They generally have a greater ability to deal with pain.

Prolactin

Prolactin will make sure that the lactating mother will continue to produce milk. All species have it.

Prolactin will program the gland cells in the breast to continue milk production even if there is dehydration, or stress known to induce dehydration. It will program the gland cells to regenerate and increase in quantity. Remember that although we concentrate on the solid composition of the milk, its water content is of equal importance to the growing fetus. Every time a cell gives rise to a daughter cell, 75 percent or more of its volume has to be filled with water. When water is brought to the area, the cells are able to access its other dissolved contents.

It has been shown in mice that increased prolactin production will cause mammary tumors. Medical scientists propose that chronic dehydration in the human body is a causative factor for tumor production. The relationship between stress, age-related chronic dehydration, persistent prolactin secretion, and inflammation of the glandular tissue in the breast should be carefully evaluated. A regular adjustment to the daily water intake in women - particularly when confronting stresses of everyday life - will at least serve as a preventive measure against possible development of stress-induced breast cancer.

Growth Hormone

Growth hormone has much similarity to prolactin. This hormone is also made in the placenta and stored in the amniotic fluid surrounding the fetus. In short, this hormone has a mammotrophic action. It makes the breast glands and ducts grow.

Cortisone

Cortisone will initiate mobilization of stored energies and raw materials. Fat is broken down into fatty acids to be converted into energy. Proteins are once again broken down into the basic amino acids for the formation of extra neurotransmitters, new proteins, and some special amino acids to be used by the muscles.

Under the influence of cortisone, the body continues to feed off itself. The effect of cortisone is designed to provide emergency raw materials for the production of essential proteins and neurotransmitters. Continued catabolic breakdown develops cumulative damage. It is this phenomenon that produces the damage associated with stress.

Vasopressin

Vasopressin regulates the selective flow of water into some cells of the body. It also causes a constriction of the capillaries it activates. As its name implies, it causes vasoconstriction. It is produced in the pituitary gland and secreted into the circulation. While it may constrict the blood vessels, some vital cells possess receiving points (receptors) for this hormone. Depending on the hierarchy of their importance, some cells appear to possess more vasopressin receptors than others.

The cell membrane - the protective covering of cell architecture - is naturally designed in two layers. Tuning fork-like solid hydrocarbon bricks are held together by the adhesive property of water. In between the two layers there is a connecting passageway where enzymes travel, selectively react together, and cause a desired action within the cell. This waterway works very much like a moat or beltway, except that it is a water-filled beltway and everything has to float in it.

When there is sufficient water to fill the space, the moat fills and water will also cross into the cell. Should the rate of water flow into the cell become insufficient the cell functions may become affected. To safeguard against such a possible catastrophic situation, nature has designed a magnificent mechanism for the creation of water filters through the membrane. The vasopressin receptor converts to a showerhead structure when vasopressin hormone reaches the cell membrane and fuses with its specially designed receptor.

The important cells manufacture the vasopressin receptor in greater quantity. Vasopressin is one of the hormones involved in the rationing and distribution of water according to a priority mechanism when there is dehydration.

The nerve cells seem to exercise their priority by manufacturing more vasopressin receptors than other tissue cells. They need to keep the waterways in their nerves fully functional. To make sure the water can pass through these tiny holes which only allow the passage of one water molecule at a time, vasopressin also has the property of causing vasoconstriction and thereby a squeeze on the fluid volume in the region.

Thus, the hypertensive property of the neurotransmitter vasopressin - better known as a hormone - is needed to bring about a steady filtration of water into the cells, but only when the free flow and direct diffusion of water through the cell membrane is insufficient.

High Blood Pressure

High blood pressure (essentially hypertension) is an adaptive process to a gross body water deficiency.

Vessels of the body have been designed to cope with fluctuation of their blood volume and tissue requirements, by an opening and closing response mechanism. When the total fluid volume in the body is decreased, the main vessels also have to decrease their aperture (close their lumen): otherwise there would not be enough fluid to fill all the space allocated to blood volume. Without adjustment to the water volume by the blood vessels, gases would separate from the blood and fill the space, causing gas locks.

Shunting of blood circulation is a normal routine. When we eat, most of the circulation is directed into the intestinal tract. The way this is done is by closing some capillary circulation elsewhere. When we eat, more capillaries are opened in the gastrointestinal tract and fewer are open in the major muscle systems. Only areas where activity places a more urgent demand on the circulatory systems will be kept fully open for the passage of blood. In other words, it is the blood-holding capacity of the capillary bed that determines the direction and the rate of flow to any site at a given time.

This process is naturally designed to cope with any priority work without the burden of maintaining an excess fluid volume in the body. When the act of digestion has taken place and less blood is needed in the gastrointestinal region, the circulation to the other areas will open more easily. In a most indirect way, this is why we feel less active immediately after a meal and ready for action after some time has passed.

In short, there is a mechanism to establish a priority for circulating blood to any given area - some capillaries open and others close. The order is determined according to importance of function. The brain, lungs, liver, kidneys, and glands take priority over muscles, bones, and the skin - unless a different priority is programmed into the system. This will happen if a continued demand on any part of the body will influence the extent of blood circulation in another, such as muscle development through regular exercise.

Water Shortage: Potential for Hypertension

When a person does not drink enough water to serve all the needs of the body, cells become dehydrated and lose water to circulation. The capillary beds in some areas will have to close so that some of the slack in capacity is adjusted. In water shortage and body drought, 66 percent is taken from the water volume normally held inside the cells; 26 percent is taken from the volume held outside the cells, and 8 percent is taken from blood volume. There is no alternative for the blood vessels other than closing their lumen to cope with the loss in blood volume. This process begins by closing some capillaries in the less-active areas. The deficient quantity must either come from outside or be taken from another part of the body.

It is the extent of capillary bed activity throughout the body that will ultimately determine the volume of circulation blood. The more the muscles are exercised, the more their capillaries will open and hold a greater volume of blood within the circulation reserves. This is the reason why exercise is a most important component for physiological adjustments in those suffering from hypertension. This is one aspect of the physiology of hypertension. The capillary bed must remain open and full, and offer no resistance to blood circulation. When the capillary bed is closed and offers resistance, only an increased force behind the circulating blood will ensure the passage of fluids through the system.

Another reason why the capillary bed may become selectively closed when there is a shortage of water in the body is because water regulates the volume of a cell from inside. Salt regulates the amount of water that is held outside the cells. There is a very delicate balancing process in the design of the body in the way it maintains its composition of blood at the expense of fluctuating the water content in some cells of the body. When there is a shortage of water, some cells will go without a portion of their normal needs and others will get a predetermined rationed amount to maintain function (as explained, the mechanism involves water filtration through the cell membrane). However, the blood will normally retain the consistency of its composition. It must do so to keep the normal composition of elements reaching the vital centers.

This is where the current perception of solutes needs to be changed. It bases all assessments and evaluations of body functions on the solid content of blood and does not recognize the comparative dehydration of some other parts of the body. Blood tests can appear normal and yet the small capillaries of the heart and the brain may be exposed to a gradual damage caused by even slight dehydration over an extended time.

When thirst sensation is lost (or the other signals of dehydration are not recognized), and less water is taken than the daily requirement, the shutting down of some vascular beds is the only natural alternative to keep blood vessels full.

The question is, how long can the body go on like this? The answer is, long enough to ultimately become very ill and die. Unless we change our perception, begin to recognize the problems associated with water metabolism disturbances in the human body and its other thirst signals, chronic dehydration will continue to be a neglected factor in the prevention and development of disease.

The operating mechanisms for adaptation to dehydration, which will climax into vasoconstriction, are the same as mentioned for stress. Namely, the continued actions of vasopressin and the R.A. System (Renin-Agiotensin System) are responsible for establishing the necessary adaptation to dehydration. They force a vascular bed reduction and increase pressure to sequence the system for showerhead water filtration into the cells in priority organs. Do not forget, dehydration is a major stressor of the human body.

Sodium is Not the Cause of Hypertension and Diuretics Worsen the Condition

Hypertension should be treated with an increase in daily water intake. The present way of treating hypertension with medication only is neglecting to treat the origin resulting in other side effects.

There is a sensitivity of design attached to sodium retention in the body. To assume this to be the cause of hypertension is inaccurate and stems from insufficient knowledge of the water regulatory mechanisms in the human body. When diuretics are given to get rid of sodium, the body becomes more dehydrated. The dry mouth level of dehydration is typical; a symptom as already explained is an advanced level of dehydration. Diuretics do not cure hypertension; they cause the body to attempt to retain more salt and water absorption - however, never enough to correct the problem. This leads to additional symptoms and new medications in a futile attempt to treat the symptoms rather than correct the cause.

Measuring Blood Pressure

There are two little known problems that occur when a patient is tested using the standard cuff method that should be included here. The anxiety associated with having hypertension will automatically affect the person at examination time. Medical readings of the instruments may not reflect the true, natural and normal blood pressure. It can happen the patient has a high reading, whereas the person may only have an instant of clinic anxiety.

The other important but less-known problem occurs when the cuff is inflated well above the systolic reading and then the air released out until the pulse is heard.

Every large (and possibly small) artery has a companion nerve that is there to monitor its flow of blood through the vessel. With the loss of pressure beyond the cuff that is now inflated to very high levels, the process of pressure opening of the obstruction in the arteries will be triggered. By the time the pressure in the cuff is lowered to read the pulsation level, the recording of an artificially induced higher blood pressure will become unavoidable. Unfortunately, the measurement of hypertension is so arbitrary (and based on the diastolic level) that a minor error in assessment may label a person hypertensive.

Water by itself is the best natural diuretic. A person who has hypertension and produces adequate urine, and increases their daily water intake, will not need to take any diuretics. If prolonged hypertension producing dehydration has also caused heart complications, water intake should be gradually increased so that fluid collection in the body is not excessive and unmanageable -proportionate to sodium retention, which will be elevated as explained above.

Water - How When and Why

Your body needs a minimum of six to eight 8-ounce glasses of water a day.

Alcohol, coffee, tea, and caffeine-containing beverages do not count as water.

Typically, the acquired taste for these drinks avoid water, the other problem is that whereas water is easily available, the other drinks are not. The author recommends that bottled water always be available in the work place, home, and carried in the car when travelling.

1. The best times to drink water are (as clinically observed in peptic ulcer disease): one glass 2 and hour before taking food -breakfast, lunch and dinner - and a similar amount 22 hours after each meal - 6 glasses.

2. This is the very minimum amount of water your body needs. One more glass of water should be taken around the heaviest meal and another before going to bed.

3. Thirst should be satisfied at all times. With increase in water intake, the thirst mechanism becomes more efficient.

4. A good habit is to always see that you have a bottle with you.

5. Adjusting water intake to mealtimes prevents the blood from becoming concentrated as a result of food intake. When the blood becomes concentrated, it draws water from cells in the surrounding area.

6. Water is the cheapest form of healing to a dehydrated body. As dehydration will in time result in one of

the many diseases, a well-regulated and constantly alert attention to daily water intake will prevent the emergence of most of the major diseases we have come to fear in our modern society.

7. When cost is a factor, tap water is permissible if the water is drawn off into a glass pot that has no Teflon or similar lining and allowed to stand over night. This will allow the chemical chlorine to evaporate. However this is only when there is proof of its not being contaminated with chemicals and heavy metals such as lead. Chlorine kills bacteria but is a toxic chemical and should be avoided directly from the tap.

8. The bottled water in supermarkets is usually sterilized by the addition of ozone at the time of bottling. Ozone, or super oxygen, has a bacteria killing property, and a good alternative source of supply.

Water Therapy and Oncology

The examples above emphasize that many symptoms, illness and disease have their origin in the development of dehydration. Clearly, the person who has developed dehydration is more vulnerable to cancer. Experience with thousands of cancer patients has presented evidence of sudden weight loss of 10-30lbs during the advanced stage or at the time of diagnosis.

This is why daily parenteral nutrition intravenous therapy is so important and should begin immediately as a matter of urgency following a diagnosis of the disease.

1. When the intervention of oncology is justified as being necessary to slow the activity and

development of the cancer, a well hydrated body will deliver chemotherapy more effectively into the cellular system at affected sites.

2. This makes a good case for immediate parenteral intravenous therapy and water intake.

3. In this book the emphasis is the impact of stress in the development of the disease. As demonstrated in this chapter dehydration is a constant source of stress. Whereas oncological intervention can be more effective as may be determined by the level of hydration, the healing potential during post-therapy must focus on reducing stress and support healing in every way to maximize recovery.

4. Stress, particularly sustained stress, accelerates catabolic damage leading to favorable conditions for the acceleration of the disease. Dehydration will therefore reduce the effectiveness of chemotherapy and interfere with recovery.

5. Adequate water will more effectively pass out chemotherapy where not needed, reducing the side effects. In this process, chemotherapy is allowed to do its work at target sites and pass out in a diluted less toxic form - especially important for the liver and kidney organs.

6. Elevated water induces more leucocyte activity, healthier plasma and hemoglobin and platelet aggregation, frequently a problem during chemotherapy.

7. Enhancing the potential level of hydration and the delivery of electrolyte fluid and water-soluble nutrients intravenously and by mouth must be a priority to maximize recovery.

Cautionary Notes

There are a number of pathological conditions such as diabetes, kidney disease, Addison's disease, thyroid, pituitary, as well as physical damage (open wounds), burns and other conditions that include diarrhea, use of diuretics, high fever and excessive perspiration that require special medical management. To this list should also be included conditions of severe stress as in shock and conditions of self-imposed or environmental impact resulting in severe electrolyte imbalances. Changes that relate to oxygen and oxygenation affecting the lungs as in breathing will also result in severe alterations that require medical management.

Acid base balance or pH also described as alkalosis (elevated pH) or acidosis (low pH - pH 7 is neutral; above 7 alkalinity increases and below 7 acidity increases). In the presence of acidosis, water tends to go from the extracellular fluid into the cells because of increased concentration of osmotically active components within the cells; this tends to accentuate the extracellular dehydration that develops. If alkalosis is present water tends to go from the cells to the extracellular compartment because of decreased concentration of osmotically active components within the cell; this tends to accentuate the edema that follows.

Chapter 6
Oxygen, Ozone and Youthful Aging

The Importance of Oxygen

Of all the chemical elements, oxygen is the most vital to the human body. We would survive for only minutes without oxygen. Oxygen is the life-giving, life-sustaining element. Approximately 90% of the body's energy is created by oxygen. Nearly all of the body's activities, from brain function to elimination, are regulated by oxygen. The ability to think, feel and act is derived from the basic energy supplied by oxygen.

However, most important is that the action of oxygen with minerals and water is the power energy that drives all body energy systems.

The only way to truly optimize health is to ensure complete cellular oxygenation together with adequate supply of minerals and water. Every one of the body's trillions of cells demands oxygen for proper function.

Oxygen is directly interrelated with minerals in several cellular, biochemical and biological systems. Whereas minerals cannot function without oxygen, oxygen cannot function without minerals.

This oxygen-energy cycle has become critically important today, more than at any time in human history, because of the sudden and unnatural decrease in atmospheric oxygen.

We have described the problem with depleted soils. When added to the problem of depleting oxygen, it is no wonder human illness, disease and deaths continue to escalate.

There are many causes for this decrease in atmospheric oxygen such as deforestation, auto and industrial pollution, devitalized soil, volcanic eruptions and so on. It has been estimated that the air breathed by our distant ancestors contained approximately 50% oxygen. Two hundred years ago, the air was composed of 38% oxygen and 1% carbon dioxide. The level measured by Swiss scientist in 1945-1946 was 22%. They have been carefully monitoring it ever since. The most recent measurement was 19% with more than 25% carbon dioxide. In our major cities the oxygen level can be lower than 10%!

It is clearly of the utmost importance that we begin to significantly increase our intake of oxygen.

Research by European doctors over several decades has proven conclusively that hyper-oxygenation of the blood through various modalities can restore vibrant health and slow or even reverse the aging process. Even advanced states of disease respond rapidly to this treatment.

Like minerals, oxygen is another seriously neglected subjected. The author includes information describing other dimensions of oxygen therapy used to treat illness and disease that should be of interest to all readers.

The Oxidation Process

Oxidation is a term used to describe the complex process of oxygen combining with various elements in the body to reduce or oxidize them for various purposes (similar to spark plugs igniting fuel to produce energy and releasing poisonous fumes out the exhaust). Oxidation is the essential factor in healthy metabolic function, better circulation, assimilation, digestion and elimination. The oxidation process is responsible for purifying the blood, keeping it free from toxic cellular waste accumulation. Adequate oxygen allows the body to recuperate during sleep, strengthening the immune system. Oxygen calms and renews the nervous system.

Proper oxidation makes the difference between health and a disease state. In *Oxidation Catalyst,* an article written for the *Journal of the American Association of Physicians,* Dr. W. Spencer Way writes:

"Internal respiration is the exchange of oxygen for carbon dioxide which takes place at the individual cell level. Without this, normal metabolism cannot take place, since it is the oxidation of the nutritional elements, which makes for their complete assimilation by the cell. Likewise, oxidation of the waste products of the cell metabolism makes possible their complete elimination."

As we have learned in previous chapters, the presence of waste products and toxins deplete minerals. Minerals work to alkalize the acids to balance critical pH.

Insufficient oxygen means insufficient biological energy that can result in anything from mild fatigue to life-threatening illness.

Dr. Otto Warburg, twice a Nobel Laureate, was awarded the Nobel Prize in 1931 for discovering the cause of cancer. He said, A*for cancer there is only one prime cause*Y *the replacement of the oxygen respiration in normal cells by the fermentation of sugar.* In other words, the growth of cancer cells is initiated by a relative lack of oxygen. Furthermore, cancer cells cannot live in an oxygen-rich environment.

Dr. Harry Goldblatt, who published his findings in The Journal of Experimental Medicine in 1953, continued this research. His research concluded that a lack of oxygen plays a major role in causing cells to become cancerous.

Dr. Albert Wahl stated: "Disease is due to a deficiency in the oxidation process of the body, leading to an accumulation of toxins. These toxins ordinarily are burned in the normal metabolic functioning." Proper oxidation contributes to a correction of disorders in the body. The cause of cancer can be removed by oxidizing body toxins.

Dr. Wendell Hendricks of the Hendricks Research Foundation wrote: "Cancer is a condition within the body wherein oxidation has become so depleted that the body cells have degenerated beyond physiological control. This depleting action may be the result of long-standing virus infection or allergies. The body becomes so overwhelmed with toxins that it sets up a natural defense in the form of a tumor mass to harbor these poisons, removing them from circulation within the body."

Dr. Steven Levine has stated it most emphatically: "Hypoxia, or lack of oxygen in the tissues, is the fundamental cause for all degenerative disease."

(Antioxidant Adaptions: Its Role in Free Radical Pathology, 1985). When the body is supplied with sufficient oxygen it will produce enough energy to ensure ideal metabolic functioning with complete elimination of accumulated toxins. Thus a state of natural immunity is obtained.

Oxygen and Ozone

While it has long been suspected that oxygen is the missing link for the healing of disease, this cannot always be directly achieved by oxygen in its O2 form. There is, however, another form of pure oxygen that is able to quickly restore proper oxidative, metabolic and immune function, even with patients wherein these functions have been severely compromised.

What Is Ozone?

Ozone, often referred to as "activated oxygen" represented chemically as O3, is pure elemental oxygen but with three atoms instead of the usual two atoms found in the oxygen that we breathe.

Ozone is naturally generated when ultraviolet light from the sun combines with oxygen in the upper atmosphere. Ozone is also created naturally through high-voltage electrical discharge such as lightning. Ozone is that fresh, clean scent in the air after a storm.

Ozone is as essential to our lives as the air we breathe. It purifies the lower atmosphere by combining with dangerous hydrocarbons, reducing them to harmless carbon dioxide and water and shields us from deadly radiation in the upper atmosphere by forming the much-talked-about ozone layer. The ancient Hebrews had an intuitive sense of the importance of ozone, referring to it as the breath of God.

Ozone has been employed as a safe effective water purifier for more than a century. It rapidly destroys viruses, bacteria and fungi as well as spores, molds, cysts and yeast. It also oxidizes chemicals and pollutants including fluorine, chlorine and THMs yielding crystal pure, sterile water.

Ozone is the second most powerful disinfectant known. Ozone kills bacterial and viral pathogens such as E. Coli 3,125 times faster than chlorine and without the carcinogenic effects. There are currently several thousand water treatment plants worldwide using ozone to purify their water resources.

Why Ozone Therapy?

Ozone is effective in the living body much the same way as it is in water purifying applications, as the body itself is composed of 70% water. Scientific studies have proven that ozone introduced into the body in repeated doses inactivates viruses, bacteria, fungi and protozoa in diseased cells while enhancing the terrain of healthy cells, improving their function.

Ozone therapy has been used in this century to kill bacteria, fungi and viruses in the body for more than 75 years. In another study, polio virus was exposed to .21 mg/liter of ozone. After 30 seconds, 99% of the viruses were inactivated. In another study, cancer cell growth inhibition was 90% when exposed to only .8 ppm (parts per million) of ozone.

Ozone therapy has been in use by hundreds of West German doctors who claim in numerous clinical studies that they are able to inactivate AIDS and other viruses as well as cancer through ozone therapy.

Remarkably enough, by 1991 in the U.S. more than 300 AIDS victims had been brought to HIV negative status and were living normal, healthy lives after using ozone therapy. These ozone treatments were administered by a handful of M.D.s, working underground at the risk of their livelihood.

HIV (along with cancer) is mistakenly viewed by the general public to be a death sentence, while ozone therapy remains either misunderstood or unknown. This is so despite the valiant efforts of informed researchers and impassioned advocates of ozone therapy to inform and report case studies especially to those who need to experience its benefits.

Side Effects from Ozone Therapy

Probably the most comforting aspect of ozone therapy is its unmatched safety and freedom from unwanted side effects.

In Germany, where ozone therapy has been accepted for many years, 644 ozone therapists were surveyed. They reported on a total of 384,775 patients, who as a group received 5,579,238 ozone treatments. Only 39 incidents of any side effect had occurred, and these were typically minor irritations of a temporary nature.

The side effects ratio of ozone therapy was thus .0007% - only 39 known side effects in more than five and a half *million* treatments!

In contrast, the side effect rate of *FDA-approved* pharmaceutical drugs in the U.S. is shocking. Figures released by the government itself show approximately *140,000 deaths annually*, with millions more suffering impaired function and broken lives - all this from FDA approved drug therapy. An unrelenting figure - more than 22 times the number of American soldiers killed during the entire Vietnam War!

How Ozone Therapy Works

This section adapted from a book *What You Should Know about Oxygen and Ozone* is included to present information considered to be helpful in further understanding of the oxygen in the cell chemistry.

In each reproducing cell of our bodies there exist two intertwined substances known as RNA and DNA B the helix form discovered by Crick and Watson. They are encoded with the genetic or blueprint for the entire body.

Viruses *are not* cells. They are *either* RNA or DNA genetic material, not both. Since they have only half of the required genetic material, they cannot reproduce on their own.

As a result of poor nutrition and/or environmental stress, normal cells become diseased. These cells develop insufficient enzyme protection in their outer layer and allow viruses to penetrate them. The viruses attach themselves to the inner RNA or DNA of these host cells and use this genetic material to multiply themselves. As these viruses multiply, their metabolic waste begins to overwhelm the body's ability to eliminate it, resulting in illness.

Outside of their host cell viruses are inert. They are hiding out in the cells and must be uncovered *within* the cells in order to be destroyed.

This is where the amazing property of ozone to invade diseased cells, uncovering and destroying viruses, is so effective. Ozone, because it possesses that third atom of oxygen, is electrophilic. It is a radical that seeks to balance itself electrically with other material with a corresponding unbalanced charge. Diseased cells, viruses, harmful bacteria and other pathogens carry such a charge, and so attract ozone and its by-products.

When ozone is introduced into the blood, it immediately begins reacting with these types of oxidizable substrates. If all the different reactants are considered, there may be 10,000 or more different ozone reactant products occurring in minute, homeopathic amounts.

These reactants kill the viruses, bacteria and fungi of macrophages, microphages and blood platelets through a mechanism called peroxide burst. In addition the metabolic waste products of these organisms are oxidized and an oxygen-rich environment is provided in which healthy cells can thrive.

In some patients, ozone treatment brings about a a healing crisis that simulates milder versions of any hidden but still significant disease process that has not been completely resolved, including allergies, drug toxicity, environmental pollution, old viral, bacterial or fungal infections or even the consequences of physical traumas and other conditions.

After the healing crisis is allowed to complete its cycle, these conditions resolve and the patient reaches a new level of well being that was previously unattainable.

It is important to note that normal, healthy cells cannot react with ozone or its by-products. Because they possess a balanced electrical charge and strong enzyme systems, they are not visible. The obvious beauty of this situation is that ozone, therefore, naturally targets only diseased cells and pathogens. Repeated applications of ozone are necessary because viruses and some forms of anaerobic bacteria are more or less susceptible to ozone at different stages of their life cycles. As an ozone reaction winds down, a new one should be introduced to react with any viruses left over from the previous treatment, and so forth.

Types of Ozone Therapy

There are currently several methods used to generate ozone for therapeutic use. However such information is described in the book by the author referred to earlier.

Self Administered Ozone External Gaseous Application:

Recent developments utilize a canvas or suitable plastic body suit, enclosing the limbs and torso of the patient. The ozone/oxygen mixture is introduced through a tube for up to 30 minutes. This is a comfortable and effective form of ozone therapy.

Other methods of gaseous ozone applications involve the creative use of various shapes of plastic containers for direct administration of ozone to affected areas. This method is especially affective in the case of trauma from injuries burns, infections and gangrene.

Ozonated Water:

Ozone is approximately ten times more soluble in water than oxygen. Mixed in water, the half-life of ozone is nine to ten hours and may be as much as doubled in refrigerated water. Ozonated water can be used orally for periodontal disease, halitosis, thrush and so forth. Taken internally, ozonated water is useful in cases of gastritis and gastric carcinoma. Used as a douche or retentive enema, ozonated water is useful in many conditions including chronic intestinal inflammations or bladder infections.

Ozone Ointment:

Highly concentrated, ozonated olive oil provides a method of long-term, low dose exposure of ozone and beneficial lipid peroxides to tissues. Used topically, it is surprisingly effective against ulcers, burns, cuts and even headache sites.

Balneotherapy:

Ozone bubbled into warm baths provides a wonderfully rejuvenating effect, enhancing circulation and balancing skin pH. Clinically it is used to provide stimulation of local circulation and disinfectant action in peripheral circulatory disorders and various dermatological conditions (eczema, ulcers, etc.)

Results of Ozone Therapy

Before outlining the result of ozone therapy in pathological conditions, it bears mentioning that ozone can be used quite successfully as a preventive health tool.

As stated earlier, we all live in a state of chronic oxygen debt or hypoxia because of various environmental factors that add up to dangerously reduced atmospheric oxygen levels. Successful genetic adaptation to this condition would take thousand of years or more. The only short-term answer is oxygenation therapy to *maintain* health.

Regular use of ozone therapy strengthens the immune system by enhancing circulation, providing an oxygen-rich environment for cellular rejuvenation, cleansing the blood of impurities, clearing plaque from the arteries, optimizing the acid/alkaline balance of the body, improving nutrient assimilation and by removing putrefactive deposits from the intestines and colon.

These and many other beneficial results of ozone therapy make it the ideal tool for rejuvenation and life extension and perhaps the most effective means for reversing the aging process.

What follows is a brief list of conditions that have been effectively treated with ozone therapy. References are included wherever possible. Because of the lack of acceptance of ozone therapy by orthodox medicine, clinical trials and double-blind studies are relatively scarce.

Candida and Epstein-Barr

These conditions are mentioned together because of their similarities. They are both chronic, apparently incurable and have recently been implicated in widespread unexplained ailments that affect millions of Americans with fatigue, depression and a variety of other symptoms. The fungicidal properties of ozone make it highly effective in the treatment of candida, both local and systematic.

The Epstein-Barr virus has been blamed for the mysterious chronic fatigue syndrome (referred to as ME in Europe). Largely considered by the medical establishment to be incurable at best and a phantom condition at worst, Epstein-Barr, like any other virus, is highly susceptible to the effects of ozone therapy.

For some research on Candida, please see *Effect of Ozone on the Survivability of Candida Utilis Cells*. Navuk et al., 1981 and *Fungi Growth and Sporulation after a Single Treatment of Spores with Ozone*. Mikol Fitopatol, 1982. And some research data on Epstein-Barr from the 1989 International Ozone Association World Congress: AIn chronic viral infections B cytomegalic, Epstein-Barr and Retroviridae (AIDS) among others B blood ozonation performed in viremic cycles or in periods of clinical exacerbation may, through direct action, through the production of co-factors inhibitory to viral replication or through modification of immune function, be a tool in inducing viral quiescence.

AIDS

AIDS is a virus and ozone has been proven in countless studies to be highly virucidal. In 1983, an international group of medical doctors meeting in Washington, D.C. for the VI World Ozone Conference, reported on their successful use of ozone therapy against the AIDS virus in their published proceedings.

In 1986, Dr. Alexander Preuss of Stuttgart, Germany issued a 39-page report on the successful result of his use of ozone therapy in 8 advanced cases of AIDS. The results were published in the scientific journal Raum & Zeit.

In 1987, Dr. Horst Kief of Heidelberg, Germany announced the successful treatments of 3 AIDS patients brought from Stage 8 back to Stage 1 at his clinic using ozone. He stated: Ayou can kill the AIDS virus with ozone therapy with no side effect. He reported that T-cell counts went from 300 up to 1500.

In 1989, Dr. George Perez, Director of Virology at Saint Michael's Medical Center in Newark, N.J. undertook a 30-day study of 5 AIDS patients using ozone. The result of "p24 test" showed massive viral destruction (a p24 test may be used to detect early HIV infection and to screen donated blood for HIV). The tests were cancelled, however, due to political pressure.

In 1990, Dr. Michael Carpendale, of the Veterans Administration Hospital in San Francisco, along with Dr. Joel Freeberg, of the University of California Medical School in San Francisco, jointly published a medical paper: *Ozone Inactivates HIV at Non-Cytotoxic Concentrations.*

In 1991, Dr. Susan Lark, M.D. of Los Altos, California, published a clinical results paper entitled: *Ozone and Its Uses In Medical Therapy.* After 10 years of research she stated, "I have found ozone/oxygen therapy to be one of the most powerful and effective therapeutic modalities I have ever worked with."

Herpes

There are number of scientific studies and papers documenting excellent results in the treatment of Herpes Simplex and Zoster with ozone therapy. It is reported that when an attack is in progress, treatment on a daily basis for 7-10 days causes a complete disappearance of symptoms. If treatments are continued for three to six weeks on a daily basis, whether symptoms are present or not, the virus can be eradicated from the patient's system. Some published results of ozone treatment of herpes include: *Ozone Vs Hepatitis and Herpes B The Choice,* Dr. Heinz Konrad, Brazil and *Ozone as Therapy in Herpes Simplex and Herpes Zoster,* Dr.K. Kattasi, et al (O.I.M.T.).

Hepatitis

In addition to the study mentioned just above, successful treatment of hepatitis with ozone was reported in many studies including the following: *The successful treatment of Viral Hepatitis with Ozone/ Oxygen Mixture,* by Dr. Kartaut Dorstewits and *Study of Chronic Hepatitis and Ozone Therapy,* by Dr. Horst Kief.

Cancer

Cancer cells have disturbed metabolisms. Nobel prize winner, Dr. Otto Warburg discovered back in 1925 that cancer cells cannot survive in the presence of oxygen. There are numerous scientific and anecdotal reports of effective treatment of cancer with ozone.

Dr. Gerard V. Sunned, M.D. stated in *Ozone in Medicine: Overview and Future Directions:* Lung carcinoma, adenocarcinoma, breast adenocarcinoma, uterine carcinosarcoma and endometrial carcinoma showed 40-90% growth inhibition depending on the concentration of ozone used.

Other references include: *The use of Ozone in Medicine,* Haug, New York, 1987 by Drs S. Rilling and R. Viebahn; *Ozone Application in Cancer Cases,* Dr. Joachim Varro; *Effects of Ozone/Oxygen Gas Mixture Injected into the Mammary Carcinoma of Mice,* Dr. Migdalia Arnan; *Successful Treatment of Neoplasm in Mice with Ozone/ Oxygen Mixture,* by Dr. Andrija Poharich; *Biochemical Reaction of an Ozone/Oxygen Mixture on Tumor Tissue,* by Dr. Joseph Washutt; and *Ozone Selectively Inhibits Growth of Human Cancer Cells,* published in Science

1980; 209; 931-933 by J. Sweet, MS Kao, D. Lee and W Hagar.

M.S., Alzheimer's, Parkinson's

Recent studies by Russian and French doctors have shown dramatic results in the treatment of Alzheimer's with ozone therapy. One reason is that it has been found that the principle cause of Alzheimer's is aluminum toxicity in the brain and ozone is recognized for its ability to precipitate aluminum.

In a similar vein, German doctors have had success with Parkinson's disease and Multiple Sclerosis as well as other neurological diseases.

In the case of M.S., it has become increasingly accepted that the cause of M.S. is a somewhat rare corona virus that demyelinates nerve coatings. Again, ozone is highly virucidal and therefore effective in conditions of this type. In another book by the author *Beyond ByPass and Chelation for Heart and Cardiovascular Disease*, it describes the success of the combined treatment of chelation and ozone use to remove mercury resulting from toxic dentistry.

Arthritis

Because of its immediate and highly beneficial effects on circulation, ozone therapy is naturally effective in the treatment of arthritis. Researchers Ed McCabe in his book Oxygen Therapies, recounts clinical work he had witnessed in Mexico: "Arthritis was usually treated every other day, and within three days there was significant reduction of pain, and by the end of the patient's stay, deformed joints were reduced as a matter a course."

In *The Use of Ozone in Medicine*, German doctors Rilling and Viebahn describe the specific protocol used successfully in arthritis, referring to the numerous papers published on the subject by Dr. H. Wolff.

Heart and Arterial Disease

The results of treatment of arterial, heart and cholesterol problems with ozone have been reported in numerous scientific journals.

Among the more prominent are the following: *Peripheral Arterial Circulation Disorders,* by Dr. Ottaker Rokitansky; *Ozone Therapy in Coronary Heart Disease,* by Dr. J. Hofmann; *Oxygen Arterial Pressure Measurement During and After Ozone Therapy,* by Dr. M. Haltin; *Ozonation of Cholesterol,* by J.Gumulka, L.Smith (J. Am. Chem. Soc. 1983).

Miscellaneous other Diseases

In their book, *The Use of Ozone in Medicine,* German doctors S. Rilling and R. Viebahn report, with extensive references, on the successful use of ozone therapy in a large number of conditions, including: acne, AIDS, allergies, anal fissures, arterial circulatory disturbances, arteriosclerosis, arthritis, arthrosis, athlete's foot, bed sores, bronchial asthma, burns, cancer, cerebral sclerosis, cirrhosis of the liver, circulatory disturbances (venous and arterial), irritable colon, constipation, cystitis, dental applications, fistulae, fungus infections, gangrene, genital infections, geriatrics, hemorrhage, hepatitis, herpes genitalis, herpes labialis, herpes zoster, hypercholesterolemia, immunostimulation, joint complaints, oral disease, stomatitis, mycosis, oncological support treatment, orthopedics, osteomyelitis, Parkinson's disease, polyarthritis, radiation scars, Raynoud's disease, RES insufficiency, shingles, skin infections, thrombophlebitis, ulcus crusis, varicosis, wound healing.

This is by no means an exhaustive list of the conditions for which ozone therapy has been successfully applied. In the years that have passed since the above work was published, many advances have been made.

The Underground Use of Ozone

In the U.S. the use of ozone began to spread rapidly in the early 1990s. So much so that America can now be said to be on the leading edge of this technology. Ingenious methodologies, daring protocols and fearless individual research have resulted in an impressive body of anecdotal data.

Is Ozone A Panacea?

Although the question in some respects begs the answer, no one is truly in a position to answer it. Certainly no other healing modality that we know of has such a remarkable range of application. We, in fact, do not know the limits of ozone treatment.

However, healing is a complex process that involves a myriad of factors, not the least of which is the individual patient's willingness or desire to be healed. And perhaps, to some extent, that is where the limitation of ozone's effectiveness will lie. In that subtle area defined by an individual's belief systems.

In fairness to our many colleagues in mainstream medicine, we'd like to point out the difficult position they are put in when an enthusiastic patient reports about the wonders of ozone therapy.

The underlying basis for much of the effectiveness of ozone treatment lies in the simple principle that diseased cells and disease cannot exist in the presence of oxygen. This simple holistic concept is difficult to swallow as most medical training is based on symptom-specific treatment. And we are cautioned to regard anything that sounds like a panacea with suspicion.

But don't be deterred. Keep on getting the word out. As wider use of ozone and other affective alternative treatments occurs, their eventual acceptance by mainstream medicine will become inevitable - for the benefit of all.

The purpose is to disseminate responsible and useful information concerning these many modalities.

The hope is that wider employment of effective alternative therapies will lead to their eventual acceptance and use by mainstream medicine for the benefit of all.

Ozone therapy has been in use throughout Europe, principally in Germany, for more than 50 years. Its safety and effectiveness has been thoroughly proven. As far back as May 1983 at the VI World Ozone Conference held here in the U.S. (Washington, D.C.), medical doctors from around the world listed 33 major diseases that had been successfully treated with ozone therapy. These included AIDS, cancer, MS, Alzheimer`s and Parkinson`s.

A textbook, published in 1987 by Haug of Heidelberg entitled *The Use of Ozone in Medicine*, lists 48 diseases commonly treated with ozone and backed their research with 225 medical ozone references.

And the FDA`s official positions regarding ozone therapy? In the Federal Register 21 CFR 801.415 dated

13 February 1976 and amended 27 September 1989, the FDA pronounced: Ozone is a toxic gas with no known medical uses.

Chapter 7
Impact of Stress

Stress in all of its many forms - emotional, mental, physical - are major factors in the depletion of minerals. The more severe and prolonged or recurring the stress is, the more cumulative the consequences leading to serous illness and degenerative disease. For example:

1. Many studies report measurable changes in the pH in response to stress. Interestingly, the pH of saliva following outrage can shift the pH to a high 11.5.

2. Biochemically, the outpouring of stress hormones such as adrenaline results in severe demands on the resources depleting reserves. Such demands experienced in one hour can be equivalent to several days or weeks of damage that is difficult to restore.

3. The familiar extra pumping heart beat and racing pulse accelerating metabolic function drawing on reserves of calcium, magnesium, and potassium is well documented. Altered electrolyte balance include sodium imbalance leading to fluid retention or edema. Most women who suffer severe

menstruation are familiar with fluid retention at that time.

4. Stress can lead to such a drain on reserves as to change a normal anabolic chemistry to become instead catabolic. This catabolic chemistry attacks weak cells altering membrane protection resulting in electrolyte imbalance and cell damage. Damaged cells release toxins causing acid environment leading to degenerative conditions.

5. The damaged or weakened cell membrane enables bacteria, virus and parasites to enter the cell resulting in severe demands on the immune system. A cumulative result is a weakened immune system unable to cope with spread of infection and damage.

6. The author has witnessed a person one day in good health change the next day to be an emergency hospital condition following a severe stress experience. This can range from sudden heart attack, stroke, brain damage, fever to serious inflammatory conditions such as arthritis, neuralgia, fibromyalgia and so on. In other case experience the individual may be the victim of stress due to a suppressive personality.

A study of these victims present evidence of a severe breakdown of electrolyte balance and altered pH. Tragically these victims are subjected to medical treatment ranging from urgent heart surgery to drug therapy adding further stress. (The author examples a case of a person rushed into his center experiencing an angina attack following an altercation in the car park across the street, who recovered instantly following an injection of magnesium citrate).

The Impact of Stress in all of its Many Forms

Years of experience and thousands of studies emphasize that the origin of cancer and degenerative disease is what the author describes as a "multicausal" development.

Although the multi-casual factors are numerous and become complex, presented here in clear order are the most common of these causal factors. Most people are unaware of the constant exposure to cancer causing pollutants in the work place and at home, the impact of denatured and chemicalized food, cancer causing methods of preparing and cooking food, incorrect eating habits, and other stress inducing factors. When informed, they will want to avoid these causal factors leading to a more natural way of living and so protect themselves to maximize healing and recovery to vibrant health.

Meeting the Demands of Stress

Throughout his years of research experience, his writing, lectures and workshops the author has emphasized the fact that stress along side nutritional deficiency, environmental pollution and toxic dentistry are major factors in the development of cancer and all other degenerative disease. He has explained the interrelationship between nutritional demands during stress in its many forms. The most dramatic healing experience is seen when nutrition is successfully adjusted to meet the demands of stress. Conversely when patients are unable to cope with any attempt to meet the demands of stress, the level of healing is slow or is no longer possible.

The author has repeatedly stated that in his opinion millions of cancer patients die of malnutrition following the side effects of cancer therapy when severe nutritional demands are not met. These are aggravated by treatment known to cause nausea or loss of interest in food. Another side effect of the treatment reported by cancer patients is the loss of taste that removes the natural desire for food. Therefore this situation is particularly challenging for the cancer patient faced with oncological treatment when the demands of stress is at its most severe.

If the body's reaction to stress is understood and the diet can be adjusted accordingly, the potential to achieve health is more certain.

The patient working to achieve the most dramatic healing short of a miracle is the one who has insight into the interrelationship between stress and nutritional demands. For this reason, this chapter is the most lengthy and most important.

Stress Explained

Stress is a reaction to experience presented as we go about our lives described as disappointment, frustration, harassment, anger, jealousy, loss of a loved one, despair, fear, anxiety and a long list of emotional and physical abuse. The intensity, frequency and duration of the stress triggers hormone and many other complex responses from the body that relies on reserves and chemical exchanges to effectively cope with these challenges.

One example of a stress response familiar to everyone is the accelerated pulse and heart beat in response to unexpected shock, fear or anxiety. There is a similar response to many other experiences occurring throughout the day. Each uses reserves requiring replenishing to ensure that repeated stresses are easily dealt with.

If these reserves become inadequate or severely depleted, a back-up response mechanism triggers a corresponding breakdown of cells and tissues to meet this stress. If allowed to continue, this catabolic state, accelerates and develops a cumulative damage, a process manifesting as degenerative disease. The normal protective systems break down, including the immune system, thereby initiating the altered state manifested as cancer in its many forms, as well as all other forms of illness and disease.

When the disease is diagnosed the cancer patient is confronted with even greater stress accelerating the break down to become even more severe than before.

Other conditions that cause damage to cells are due to contact with chemicals in the environment, free radicals from food cooked in heated oils and fats, toxic metals, electromagnetic pollution, radiation, surgery and physical damage due to accident and burns. If nutrition is adequate, cells quickly repair the damage, but when rebuilding fails to keep pace with destruction, illness is accelerated.

Cumulative Damage

Disease is accelerated as a result of other multiple stresses added to those already described such as overwork, bacterial or viral infection, parasites, inadequate or restless sleep, and no exercise. Unfortunately, these examples usually lead to numerous other stresses: poor appetite, nausea, vomiting, faulty digestion, fever, pain, diarrhea, dehydration, high urinary losses of many nutrients, exposure to x-rays, and the use of drugs.

The Demands for Repair are Severe

In the same way that it requires more material for the repair of a damaged house than the upkeep of one in good condition, every nutrient is needed in larger amounts to repair a body damaged by the multiple stresses that cause disease and result from it. For example, the extensive evidence of the stress - or damage - following x-rays or the response to any one of many commonly used drugs, increases the need for protein, linoleic acid, several minerals, vitamins A, C, the anti-oxidants and all the B vitamins.

Regardless of the forms of stress, the body immediately tries to repair damage done. However, such repair depends on the generous supply of all nutrients needed to achieve this. The nutritional needs increase tremendously at the very time eating is most difficult, and a diet inadequate for a healthy individual becomes seriously inadequate for an ill person.

The Body's Reaction to Stress

The great medical genius Dr. Hans Selye, of the University of Montreal, revolutionized medical thinking with his theory, since confirmed by thousands of scientific studies, that the body reacts to every variety of stress in some way.

At the onset of stress, a tiny gland at the base of the brain, the pituitary, responds with a protective action by secreting chemical messengers, or hormones, ACTH (adrenocorticotropic hormone) and STH (somatotropic hormone). These hormones, carried in the blood to two small glands above the kidneys, the adrenals, cause the outside border of these glands, or cortex, to produce cortisone and other messenger hormones.

Although the center of these glands manufacture adrenaline, the adrenal hormones referred to throughout this book are those made by the cortex.

Flight or Fight

Alarm Reaction Stage 1

These adrenal cortex hormones quickly prepare the body to meet the emergency: proteins, at first drawn from the thymus and lymph glands, are broken down to form glucose necessary for immediate energy; the blood sugar soars and the remaining sugar is stored in the liver in the form of body starch, or glycogen, which can be instantly converted to sugar if needed; the blood pressure increases, minerals are drawn from the bones, fat is mobilized from storage deposits, an abnormal amount of sodium is retained, and many other changes take place which prepare the body for "fight or flight." These changes also make it possible to repair vital tissues by a process of robbing Peter to pay Paul. This stage, called the "alarm reaction," varies in intensity with the degree of stress.

Resistance Stage 2

If the stress continues, the body sets up a "stage of resistance" in which it repairs itself by rebuilding with all the raw materials available. When the diet is adequate, a person may go for years coping with tremendous stress with little apparent harm. Should the raw materials be insufficient to meet the needs, however, there comes a "stage of exhaustion."

Exhaustion Stage 3

Disease develops, if it has not already done so, and eventually death threatens or results.

These initial two stages of stress are characterized by constant damage and repair; most illness fall in stage three, which is reached when repair fails. Intense stress, such as surgery, a serious car accident, or severe burn, may cause a person to pass through all three stages - alarm, resistance, and exhaustion - in a single day. More often we experience repeated alarm reactions and live through hundreds of stages of resistance, one piled on top of the other, before pituitary and adrenal exhaustion threatens our lives. During every illness, however, we are in one of these three stages of stress, and to regain health, diets must be planned accordingly.

Catabolic Stress Attacks Vulnerable Sites

If stress is prolonged after the thymus and lymph glands (whose proteins are necessarily drained) have shriveled, proteins from the blood plasma, liver, kidneys, and other parts of the body are used. Stomach ulcers may occur not only because of increased production of hydrochloric acid, but also because proteins are robbed from the stomach walls. In ulcerative colitis, the destruction of protein brought about by prolonged stress literally eats away the lining of the intestine. During a single day of severe stress, the urinary loss of nitrogen has shown that the amount of body protein destroyed equals that supplied by 4 quarts of milk. Yet if such a tremendous quantity of protein can be eaten during the day, the tissues are unharmed.

In the same way that the body suffers when its proteins are necessarily stolen and not replaced, so are the bones weakened by the loss of calcium. Dozens of other destructive changes similarly occur. Increased blood pressure alone may become dangerous. It is extremely important, therefore, to learn how to protect ourselves from the ravages of stress.

In all stages of the fight or flight response there is also severe demand that drains mineral reserves. Not only calcium from the bones, but also due to the accelerated functions there is a release of hormones that uses minerals - particularly trace minerals. It is clear that there is a greater demand on minerals as the build up of metabolic function accelerates as well as when minerals counteract the acids resulting from catabolic damage. The state of exhaustion results when reserves of daily replenishment are inadequate to meet the demand.

Stress Factors

Experimental stress has been produced in animals by exposing them to loud noises, blinking lights, extreme heat or cold, rarefied air, electric shock, x-rays and other forms of radiation; by injecting into them drugs, chemicals, bacteria, or viruses; by submitting them to surgery, burns, accidents, fasting, immobility, or making them run on a treadmill to exhaustion; and by feeding them mineral oil, innumerable toxic substances, or diets deficient or excessive in one or more nutrients.

The nutritional needs of these animals invariably skyrocket at the onset of stress and remain high in comparison with those animals not submitted to such torments. Stress produced by forced exercise, giving excessive thyroid, or exposure to x-rays increases the need for all nutrients. If these increased nutritional requirements are met, little harm is done; if not, damage may be severe or even fatal.

Impact of Nutrition on the Pituitary and Adrenals

How well animals cope with stress depends to a considerable degree on their ability to produce pituitary and adrenal hormones. If the diet has been inadequate in protein, vitamin E, or the B vitamins, riboflavin (vitamin B2), pantothenic acid, or choline, and certain trace minerals, sufficient pituitary hormones cannot be produced. Vitamin E, which is more concentrated in the pituitary gland than in any other part of the body, is particularly important in preventing both the pituitary and adrenal hormones from being destroyed by oxygen.

Impact of Pantothenic Acid

The adrenal cortex is even more sensitive to dietary deprivation. A pantothenic-acid deficiency causes the glands to shrivel and to become filled with blood and dead cells; cortisone and other hormones can no longer be produced, and the many protective changes characteristic of stress do not occur. Even a slight lack of pantothenic acid causes a marked decrease in the quantity of hormones released. The pituitary, adrenal, and sex hormones are all made from cholesterol, but without pantothenic acid, cholesterol cannot be replaced in the glands after once being used up. If generous amounts of pantothenic acid are given and the deficiency has not been severe, adrenal hormones can be produced normally within 24 hours. When the deprivation has been prolonged, however, a period of repair is necessary and recovery is slow and uncertain.

Vitamins A, E, B2 Linoleic Acid and Trace Minerals

A slight deficiency of linoleic acid or vitamin A, B2, or E can also limit hormone production and cause degeneration of the adrenal cortex; hence each is as essential as pantothenic acid.

Adrenals of volunteers low in essential fatty acids produced markedly fewer hormones than when the diet was adequate. Damage resulting from such deficiencies can be quickly rectified because the adrenals need these nutrients in small amounts only. Vitamin B2 given to animals previously deficient restored the normal adrenal function. When oil supplying linoleic acid is given to rats lacking it, the production of adrenal hormones quickly increases almost 90 per cent.

Vitamin C

Although adrenal hormones can be produced without vitamin C, the need for this nutrient is tremendously increased by stress; and, if under supplied, the glands quickly hemorrhage and the output of hormones is markedly decreased. This vitamin accelerates the rate of cortisone production, appears to improve its utilization, delays its breakdown, and alleviates many of the limitations resulting from a pantothenic acid deficiency. Apparently because large amounts of vitamin C are used to detoxify harmful substances formed in the body during stress, greater-than-normal quantities are lost in the urine at this time.

Huge amounts of vitamin C appear to protect animals from every form of stress. For example, rats exposed to severe cold died unless they received massive quantities of this vitamin. Guinea pigs, exposed to the same low temperature, remained healthy when given 75 times their normal requirement of vitamin C; if allowed smaller amounts, their adrenals hemorrhaged and many animals died.

Translated into human terms, 75 times our normal daily requirement of vitamin C would be approximately 5,625 milligrams. Such a quantity seems startling, yet during severe stress it may not be excessive.

144 elderly hospitalized patients, whose adrenal glands could no longer respond normally, when stimulated with the pituitary hormone ACTH, and given 500 milligrams of vitamin C daily, had their adrenals markedly improved. Adrenal hormones in the blood and urine increased immediately. Though the patients suffered from various illnesses and their medication remained unchanged many showed marked improvement.

Intensity Determines Nutritional Requirements

Mild abnormalities may call for only a few dietary improvements, but serious illness, when stresses are piled upon stresses, causes the nutritional requirements of the entire body especially the pituitary and adrenal glands to be severe. Any deficiency becomes worse in proportion to the number, kind, and intensity of stresses. Often such large quantities of vitamin A are excreted in the urine such that any amount stored is quickly exhausted. Severe stress also causes the non-essential amino acids - those normally made in the body - to become essential because the body cannot produce them rapidly enough. To meet such nutritional demands depends on the adequacy of the diet both before and during the stress itself.

The Anti-Stress Factors

Certain vitamin-like substances called the anti-stress factors are still the subject of intense study. Details are not necessary for inclusion in this book. However their importance is clear in studies with animals fed certain foods known to be high in these anti-stress factors that demonstrate unusually surprising protective action against most types of stress, though not all.

For example, when rats are given strychnine, sulfanilamide, quinacrine hydrochloride (trade name Atabrine Hydrochloride), stilbestrol, excessive thyroid, cortisone, or aspirin, all cause harmful effects that cannot be overcome by increased amounts of any known vitamins, mineral, or other nutrient. Yet the animals are completely protected if given foods supplying the anti-stress factors. These substances also prolong the survival time of rats exposed to x-rays.

Wheat Germ

One classic study repeated many times is this anti-stress factor in wheat germ providing a remarkable resistance in animals injected with various bacteria.

Other Sources

The anti-stress factors are found in liver, nutritional yeast, and soy flour from which the oil has not been removed. Another source of anti-stress factors, different from the one in liver, is found in the pulp of green leafy vegetables. Research indicates that ill persons should work as many of these foods as possible into their daily diets.

Reaction to Stress and Disease

A symptom of an illness or even a disease is often the body's reaction to stress. Adrenal hormone, desoxycorticosterone acetate or DOC (trade names Doca Acetate and Percorten Acetate), for example, often counter balances the effects of cortisone, keeping it in check. DOC helps the body to fight infections and protects it by setting up an inflammation around bacteria and toxic substances, preventing them from spreading to surrounding tissues; thus is a boil or tubercular lesion walled off.

DOC causes blood and tissue fluids to be drawn to a damaged area, white blood cells and other defense mechanisms to be called in; although swelling, pain and fever results, the remainder of the area is protected. Thus the reaction to stress, occurring during any inflammation, becomes the illness or disease.

Such a disease is given the name of the organ involved, with the ending >tis'. Arthritis, bursitis, colitis, and nephritis among others, are spoken of as Astress diseases."

If so little cortisone can be produced that DOC is not held in check, the inflammation can get out of hand and continue year after year, as it does in arthritis, some allergies, and many diseases. On the other hand, if too little DOC can be produced or if cortisone is given as a medication, the body becomes susceptible to infections, inflammations, and damage form toxic substances.

Another adrenal hormone, aldosterone, holds salt (sodium) and water in the body, thus preventing dehydration. When it is being produced in excessive amounts during the first two stages of stress, so much water may be retained that the hands, ankles, and eyes become puffy and too much potassium is lost in the urine. Such a condition can be the cause of high blood pressure and may become a major problem during certain types of kidney and heart disease. Restricting the salt intake at such a time causes aldosterone to be excreted and prevents the loss of potassium. Taking potassium to replace the urinary losses also rectifies this situation.

Adrenals exhausted from prolonged stress are unable to produce sufficient amounts of aldosterone; too much salt and water are lost from the body, the blood pressure usually falls below normal, dehydration occurs, and potassium is withdrawn from the cells. In this case salt (sodium) rather than potassium is needed. Salt intake therefore, should be restricted during the alarm reaction, moderate during the Astage of resistance, and high if the adrenals become exhausted. Rats under prolonged stress, allowed to select their own diet and offered separate nutrients - except vitamin C which they synthesize - will particularly increase their intake of salt and pantothenic acid.

ACTH and Cortisone Therapy

There are times when ACTH or cortisone must be given, and each physician carefully weighs the many advantages against the disadvantages. Either sets up a condition coinciding to the onset of stress, accelerates the breakdown of body protein and so prevents healing, or the synthesis of new proteins causes the thymus and lymph glands to atrophy, or shrivel, and water and salt may be held in the body. A decrease of natural hormone production inhibits the synthesis of anti-bodies and white blood cells needed to fight infections, increases both the need for almost every requirement and the urinary losses of amino acids, calcium, phosphorous, potassium, all the B vitamins, vitamins A, and C.

Side Effects of ACTH

Persons being given ACTH (adrenocorticotropic hormone) or cortisone often develop stomach ulcers and severe spontaneous bruising, nose bleeds, and hemorrhages; if sugar formed from the destruction of body proteins is not used for energy, it is changed into fat, which accounts for part of the gain in weight when cortisone is taken.

Dr. Selye points out that while patients receiving cortisone may have an unusual feeling of well-being at first, they often develop high blood pressure, insomnia, infections, disturbances of the intestinal tract, and may become so depressed as to have suicidal tendencies. Such toxicity can be markedly decreased, the period of therapy shortened, and either ACTH or cortisone made more effective if the diet is extremely adequate and especially high in protein, vitamins C and E, and all the B vitamins. Much harm can result when ACTH is given unless large amounts of pantothenic acid are taken with it; supplements of vitamin C and potassium should accompany cortisone therapy.

Case Histories

Case histories report a man who had been given cortisone for three years for arthritis had suffered seven broken vertebra, which had fractured spontaneously from the pressure of his own body; also a women who had taken cortisone for three years had developed Addison's disease, or total adrenal exhaustion. These toxic effects are unnecessary but they do occur. Because of such hazards, it is preferable to allow the body to produce its own hormones whenever possible.

Filling the Demands of Stress

That adrenal exhaustion has become widespread is shown both by the millions of persons suffering from stress disease and by the number of illnesses for which physicians now give cortisone. Yet the person deficient in pantothenic acid - which seems to be most of our population - receives the same benefit from taking the vitamin as from ACTH or cortisone and with no toxic side effects. When this is combined with the anti-stress fortified drink, this response is in most cases predictable.

To meet the demands of stress - and health can never be restored until they are met - the starting point is to obtain all nutrients necessary for the production of the pituitary and adrenal hormones.

As previously mentioned quantities of protein, vitamin C, and pantothenic acid required are particularly high, however, they vary with individuals and the severity of stress. For example practitioners often recommend too little, such as 20 milligrams of pantothenic acid daily for ill persons, or as high as 15,000 milligrams, given daily for long periods (with no toxic effects) but is prohibitively expensive.

A combination of vitamins found to give excellent results that should be obtained during every illness or severe stress is described as the anti-stress formula. Because these vitamins dissolve in water, they are readily lost in the urine; hence more effective when amounts are taken frequently rather than larger quantities at one time. Vitamin B2 is essential for the synthesis of adrenal hormones, but if given alone, a vitamin B6 deficiency is produced; therefore the amounts of these two vitamins should always be kept the same. Supplements combining these are best or a capsule containing vitamin C and several B vitamins when need is increased by stress.

The Ultimate Goal

When health is once attained and further stress is recognized, the diet can be improved before serious illness occurs. If such a procedure is followed, a long and rewarding life free from disease becomes attainable.

Chapter 8
Nutrition, Diet, and Supplements

This chapter flies in the face of the establishment. There are many different models, ranging from the RDA guidelines, the dietitian's food pyramid, metabolic typing, zone diets, Atkins high protein diet, rotation diets, fasting and many others.

Americans spend billions of dollars and change their lifestyles in expectation of success based on the claims of many experts and books. Many Americans in search of the magic formula have tried several or all of the above.

The truth is that these and similar models to come will fail so long as the experience described in this book is not applied. It is unscientific to claim that one particular model will work for everyone. Firstly, this flies in the face of the evidence first presented by Roger J. Williams described as biological individuality - that is that no two individuals are the same. Furthermore, factors such as lifestyle, stress, individual past history of mental and emotional frustration, abuse and suppression, exposure to toxic environment and so on complicate the assumption of these models. A major problem with these models is the assumption that food and diets recommended deliver nutrients from a natural source of food supplying all the nutrients needed to meet the conditions necessary to achieve the claims made. This ignores the evidence that our depleted soils produce plants and animal food deficient in a number if these nutrients. It ignores the evidence that two apples from the same tree provide different amounts of nutrients. It ignores the evidence that early harvesting, storage, preparation and method of cooking can alter the nutritional value of foods recommended. Microwave cooking and deep frying actually alter natural food into toxic free radicals, it ignores the fact that processing our food has so altered nutrition and depleted nutrients, it ignores the negative impact of medications and drugs and use of antibiotics - the list is too vast to describe here! None of these factors were necessary to produce vibrant health displayed by the tribes described elsewhere.

Dr. Williams presented studies proving that vibrant health was achieved when daily diet and nutrition was balance to supply vitamins, natural oils, organic raw whole milk and eggs from free range chickens, enzymes and minerals. This was particularly so with organically grown food in rich soils. The point here is that a balanced diet of nutritious food was capable of restoring most health problems naturally and permanently with all people without the need to follow special diets described above.

The common denominator of the many cultures who live to be 135 years and older while maintaining a vigorous youth in disease free societies, is their soil being constantly replenished with mineral nutrients, most of which are missing in our soil. Except for some of the Japanese on Okinawa, all these societies live in mountainous regions. They are the Tibetans, the Hunzukuts of Northern Pakistan, the Armenian, the Georgians, the Azerbaijanis, the Vilcabamba Indians in Ecuador and the Titicacas in Peru, and a few other cultures. All their soils are replenished with mineral nutrients contained in the turbid water from melting glaciers (turbid water has sediment or foreign particles stirred up or suspended). The contained glacial-crushed minerals are so abundant that the water is white and is known as the milk of the mountains. The islands of Okinawa were built up over the years from coral reefs. Rain erodes the coral reefs producing mineral rich milk of the oceans. All of these cultures drink their water turbid. The contained dissolved minerals are so abundant that when they drink their customary four quarts each day, all of these disease-free societies violate our doctor recommended daily allowances (RDA) by massive amounts. For example, they consume 70 times the RDA of calcium, 22 times the RDA for magnesium, 18 times the RDA of potassium, 126 times the RDA of iron, 120 times the RDA of fluoride, etc. To top it off, they continue to exceed these RDA's even further by eating *food* which is rich in these minerals. They also consume RDA unacceptable amounts of trace minerals in their water while maintaining a killer diet rich in eggs, raw whole cream milk, and butter.

The Hunzukuts drink their 30 daily cups of tea, each with a large hunk of rock salt and two patties of butter. Our modern American doctors, who die prematurely, incomprehensibly recommend that you do not follow the dietary example of the youthful, energetic and disease-free 135 year old Hunzukuts. Nutrient-trained veterinarians, on the other hand, have long recognized the importance of mineral, metal and vitamin supplements, and as a result animal food is full of these supplements. For example, horse and dog food can contain as much as 60 nutrient supplements, while human food remains almost totally depleted in these life-sustaining nutrients. As long as animals are fed only animal food and not people food, they remain relatively disease-free.

In the kingdom of Hunza, the freedom from a variety of diseases and physical aliments is remarkable. Cancer, heart attacks, vascular complaints and many childhood diseases such as mumps, measles and chicken pox are unknown among them. The diet upon which these people have lived for centuries is responsible for the enviable good health they enjoy, it cannot be matched in our civilization with its depleted soil, processed food robbed of its life-giving elements, and cooking methods that effectively destroy a substantial percentage of the vitamins and trace elements that are essential to sound bodies. The United States lead the world in material progress and standards of good living, yet, in respect to the raising of truly nutritious food, it lags far behind the little kingdom of Hunza.

A Medical Opinion

In a talk to members of the American Medical Association (reported in Newsweek, June 17, 1959), Tome Douglas Spies, M.D., a recipient of the AMA Distinguished Service Award, said: AAll disease is caused by chemicals, and all disease can be cured by chemicals. All the chemicals used by the body, except for the oxygen we breathe and the water we drink, are taken in through food. If we only knew enough, all disease could be prevented and could be cured through proper nutrition.

Clearly, choice of food, daily diet and supplements has a major impact on the state of mineral balance.

Explanation of the Ionizing Process of Digestion

It is now appropriate to explain in simple terms the ionizing process that makes nutrients in the food available in a form easily transported to cells for efficient use. This explanation will also help to clarify the important selection of food for their acid and alkaline values.

The dictionary explains digestion as the process by which food is broken down mechanically and chemically in the gastrointestinal tract and converted into absorbable forms. Salts (minerals), water, and monosaccharides can be absorbed unchanged, but starches, fats, and proteins must be broken down into smaller molecules. This is brought about by enzymes, each of which acts on a specific type of food and requires a specific pH to be effective.

Hormones released by the gastrointestinal mucosa stimulate the secretion of digestive enzymes and bile influencing the motility (peristalsis) of the stomach and intestines. Starches and disaccharides are digested to monosaccharides; fats are digested to fatty acids and glycerol; proteins are digested to amino acids. During digestion, vitamins and minerals are liberated from these large organic molecules.

Although this definition assumes guidelines for a well balanced diet, it fails to explain the chemistry that goes beyond digestion that is so critical to the effective delivery and transport of nutrients made possible by ionization. In fact, without such ionization the process of digestion is incomplete.

In more technical terms the ionization of animal and plant nutrients are presented as their basic anion (negative) and cation (positive) components, so that these ions can be properly transported into the cells.

The process of ionizing plant, animal, or mineral nutrients begins with pulverizing them through chewing and the action of the stomach to expose as much of the surface as possible to water. For some nutrients, such as salt sodium chloride, the exposure to water is all that is required to initiate immediate ionization. Most nutrients however require the addition of acid to the pulverized nutrient and water mixture to effect any significant amount of ionization.

When digestion is initiated hydrochloric acid is released to lower the pH necessary to digest protein food and to neutralize high alkaline foods and drinks. This is an initial stage of a buffering system that continues throughout the numerous fluid systems in the body.

Fortunately, or by design, the digestive system is made more efficient by the fact that most food is acidic, thereby generating their own acids and thus requiring less acid from the body for total digestion.

There are several points to make:

1. There needs to be a combination of both acids and alkalies to achieve ionization of nutrients.

2. Because the body needs to have protein (amino acids) it is unwise to focus on alkaline foods only.

3. The ultimate diet will balance organically grown food selected to ensure that all of the digestive functions described are efficient.

Nutrition and Diet

Consider the following:

1. Firstly it is important to realize that food depleted of minerals (food from depleted soils or refined processed food), or with minerals missing, require that the body draw on its reserves to digest and assimilate and transport available nutrients.

2. Refined processed and microwaved food produce acids that must be neutralized by minerals.

3. Food grown in deficient soils fail to deliver minerals that have to be drawn from the pool of minerals so disturbing the natural balance. Deficiencies of these missing minerals lead to serious disease. Example is soils deficient in iodine that cause thyroid disease. Also, many studies link soils deficient in selenium to cancer.

4. It is clear that the chemicals used to protect plants against bugs and insects enter the plant and also seep into the soil. These chemicals interfere with the delicate balance of bacteria and microbes living in the soil. These toxic chemicals enter the body chemistry requiring minerals to neutralize them. These chemicals damage cells making them vulnerable to attack by parasites, bacteria and virus. They also disrupt the delicate osmotic pressure between the interior and exterior membrane.

5. Coffee, tea, carbonated drinks, alcohol, sugar deplete minerals (Coca Cola is reported to have an acid pH of 2.5).

6. Food cooked in oil and fats particularly deep fried food, fries and microwaved food are known to be

free radicals which deplete minerals. The habit of concluding a meal with a desert or coffee with sugar or alcohol exacerbates the problem further.

7. Drinking water with ice added together with food is so unnatural as to alter pH, washes foods down undigested, removes the natural defense against bacteria and parasites in the food and much more.

Criteria for selecting alkaline and acid food

1. Firstly, there is a notion that the correct approach to over acid or alkaline pH is to focus on alkaline food. Various experts present lists of food and drinks categorized as acid or alkaline recommending that the daily diet avoid acid food. As exampled in this chapter, this approach is in conflict with nature's law of balance determined by a variety of foods to ensure an efficient digestion and balanced nutrition.

2. 2. There are different interpretations presented by these experts as to which are acid or alkaline foods. To illustrate the problem the following list presents the content of so called alkaline foods:

To further complicate an evaluation of the above pH values, the digestion will alter the pH depending on factors such the HCL (hydrochloric acid) release, combination with other foods, how the food is cooked, even the mental state of the person during the meal. The point is that whereas the pH of stomach contents during digestion may be a low 1-3, ionization with fluid produces negative anions to balance pH of food as it moves along in he process of digestion.

There is a notion that the alkaline food listed is all that is necessary to correct the acid pH. There are too many other factors in the biological individuality that are in conflict with this notion.

Food	pH	Food	pH
Lemons	2.1	Beans	5.5
Apples	3.1	Bread	5.5
Grapefruit	3.1	Asparagus	5.6
Rhubarb	3.1	Potatoes	5.8
Strawberries	3.2	Butter	6.3
Raspberries	3.4	Corn	6.3
Tomatoes	4.2	Shrimp	6.9
Bananas	4.6	Water	7.0
Carrots	5.1	Egg White	7.8

Scientific Guidelines

Acid forming foods are those that:
1. Have been grown in chemically fertilized soil
2. All animal and poultry cooked meat
3. Have been subjected to processing
4. Have been subjected to extreme temperatures in cooking and freezing
5. Have been cooked or fried in heated fats and oils. This is especially so when cooked in recycled oil or margarine

6. Food cooked in a microwave
7. All sugar and sugar based food
8. Soda drinks - Coca-Cola has a pH of 2.5
9. Coffee and all caffeine containing drinks

Note: It is not only the acid pH resulting from sugar and drinks; it is the chain reaction that follows ingestion together with other food and drinks. Particularly the altered state of the balance accelerating positive acid pH cations.

Add to this list all medications and drugs.

Alkalining Food
1. All fresh uncooked vegetable salads - organic
2. All fresh fruits - organic
3. Steamed vegetables - organically grown
4. Natural spring water - do not use distilled water which has no minerals (meaning that the more distilled water, the more the body compensates further depleting reserves)
5. Green foods such as Spirulina, Wheat Grass, Chlorella
6. Sea plants including dulse and a variety of sea weeds
7. Raw whole organic whole cream milk, yogurt
8. Sprouted seeds

Therapeutic Nutrition

Therapeutic nutrition applies the principles outlined in this book in more scientific individualized form when illness and disease is presented.

Individualized therapeutic nutrition assesses biological individuality, using information provided by the individual including an extensive NutriMedical Health and Lifestyle Assessment Questionnaire. This is available in consultation with a medical doctor or licensed practitioner.

Additional Guidelines

This information describing additional guidelines is considered of special value resulting from the research experience accumulated by the author.

Eggs

Eggs are outstanding in their nutritional benefits, for they are abundant in all the essential amino acids. The yolk is rich in vitamin E, biotin, choline, inositol, vitamin A, and other sulfur-containing amino acids, that are so rare in most food. The egg white has substantial amounts of riboflavin and the complete protein albumin. Raw eggs give the highest benefits because heat has not altered the vitamin structure. Always eat the white and yolks together. All cooking must be done gently. It is particularly important not to hard boil eggs as the lecithin or cholesterol-protecting substance will be destroyed. Eggs should always be from naturally fed chickens (free range) that have not been given hormones or genetically engineered food.

The healthiest method of cooking eggs is to place them in cold clean water (not tap water) bring to the boil and then immediately switch off and allow to stand in the boiled water for 10-15 minutes. Reserve the boiled egg water and use for cooking your vegetables or soup - the reason being you will get the calcium from the eggshells.

Organic Food

Nature abounds with a vast variety of edible plants, fruit, grains, beans and so on to ensure that all essential nutrients are available. Nature is in fact telling us to plan our nutrition and diet to include a variety of food. In recent years the mounting opposition to chemicalized and processed food has spawned the development of growers and farmers producing organically grown food. Organic vegetables may have bruise spots and evidence of damage from pests. Select the best but do not be turned away from organic foods. One portion of organic food will provide a more complete range of nutrients that could not be duplicated by one hundred portions of plants grown in chemically fertilized soil.

Substitute brown rice, lentils, chick peas and other varieties of beans for the refined white rice. Studies suggest that grains and legumes are incomplete amino acids. A solution is to combine when ever possible both legumes and grains which compliment each other to form complete protein. Try combining the grains and beans in the dried form ready for soaking and cooking.

Green food is a particularly good source of minerals. So too are sprouted seeds and wheat grass. Rich source of minerals and enzymes include, Clorella, and Spirulina powders.

Salad Storage and Preparation

Salads are superior as a means of serving nutrients for good health. Try and get a wide variety of vegetables. Vegetables should always be stored in a dry, cold state - not wet! As soon as the vegetable is washed (in clean water not from the tap) it should be dried before storage. Otherwise, the water withdraws vitamins and minerals from the plant through a process called osmosis, and the benefits of good nutrition are lost. Wash and store all vegetable peelings, tops etcetera in the refrigerator until needed. The water used to wash vegetables should be saved and fed to your plants. Add fresh vegetables to soups at the very end and they will always be a little crisp. Always try to keep all food organic and use only organically grown fresh vegetables and fruit. By doing this you can have the assurance that there will be a quality cell structure, high vitamin-mineral content, and freedom from harmful sprays and inorganic fertilizers.

Salads made up of several vegetables should ideally be included twice a day. Include tomato, onion, avocado, cucumber, lettuce and other vegetables of choice. Add a dressing made with organic apple cider vinegar, flax seed oil and raw organic honey to produce a tasty salad with the added value of essential fatty acids and minerals.

Supplements

This book has described the natural synergism of all nutrients working to balance minerals, vitamins, amino acids and enzymes.

Billions of dollars are spent on supplements claiming to achieve cures for symptoms, illness and disease.

The truth is that as we move more into organic farming, the quality of organically grown food depends on the quality of the soil in which these are grown. For this reason there is a good case for supplementation. However, this should not be a haphazard selection based on claims. Consider the following:

a. All nutrients work best in a synergistic chemistry. Minerals are essential to activate enzymes, necessary to digest food, necessary for vitamins to produce energy and amino acids to build cells.

b. Whereas scientific study has determined the function of many of these individual nutrients, it is impossible to measure the correct dosages for each person. The exact science of a means to measure these nutrients to determine correct supplements is an impossible challenge complicated by a biological individuality. It follows that supplements -particularly when individual supplements are used - is guesswork. However, there are many documented studies that have successfully determined dosages to reverse disease. The best example is iodine to reverse thyroid problems.

The point here is that a knowledgeable selection of supplements is vital to avoid disturbing existing problems and correct deficiencies to balance chemistry.

Clearly the ultimate objective is to have a scientifically balanced easily absorbed supplement supplying all the minerals, vitamins, enzymes and amino acids. To my knowledge there is only one crystalloid liquid supplement that fulfills this requirement. Based on sea plants, this supplement ensures that all these nutrients are included in one formula.

The body will use this crystalloid liquid supplement far more effectively. What is not known is how much is adequate to satisfy individual needs to correct existing deficiencies.

In the case of illness and disease when it is clear that minerals will speed recovery, the above crystalloid liquid should be taken together with the homeopathic electrolyte crystalloid solution described in Chapter 2 (see *Homeopathic Formula* in the index).

Vitamin C

The author has observed that vitamin C in the ascorbate form enhances the uptake and homeostasis of minerals.

An excellent source of minerals and vitamin C is the Twins™ product ascorbate powder. Powder is made from mineral ascorbates, calcium, magnesium, zinc, manganese and potassium ascorbates. Ascorbates are easier to absorb.

The impact of vitamin C on the healing process is so dramatic that a short description is appropriate.

It is common knowledge that a few milligrams of vitamin C daily will prevent acute scurvy. What is not commonly known is the extent to which stress demands deplete vitamin C levels resulting in a number of health problems.

Symptoms may include bleeding gums, mental sluggishness, irritability, and borderline anemia. Flu and colds will be frequent, illness will be prolonged, and recovery slow.

Tissue will bruise easily, injuries will heal slowly, skin conditions and muscle tone may be poor. Kidney and bladder stones may develop. One may be susceptible to allergies. Signs of aging will occur earlier than they would if supplies of the vitamin were adequate.

When daily doses of ascorbate C are maintained in

the thousands of milligrams, these susceptibilities will usually cease. A person will then rarely contract a cold, the flu, or any bacterial or viral disorder. Infections and injuries will heal rapidly, and bruises will be mild, occurring only after the most severe blows.

Dosages in the tens of thousands of milligrams can have even more profound results. Cancers and tumors may be prevented or regressed, and lifespan may be prolonged considerably.

Wrinkling and other visible signs of aging will be delayed. Mental senility, loss of sexual libido, stooped stature, arthritic pains, and other chronic symptoms of aging will be delayed. Fragile, porous bones that fail to mend if broken are one of the greatest threats of the aged. If ascorbate C levels are high and other nutritional and hormonal factors are in order, mending will be almost as rapid at 80 or even 120, as it was at 40.

Ascorbates

Sodium ascorbate should be avoided, especially by those with high blood pressure, or on a low sodium diet. Even for a normal person, this is too much sodium if the mega-ascorbic doses suggested are taken. Sodium causes the tissues to retain water and inhibits the diuretic effects of ascorbic acid. Some bottles of tablets that are labeled vitamin C are actually sodium ascorbate. Always check the fine print on the side of the label.

The correct form of vitamin C is available as the ascorbate of essential minerals, including calcium, magnesium, zinc, manganese, and selenium. These have no acidity. Minerals as ascorbates are very easily assimilated, and the vitamin is more stable in this form. When taking these ascorbates, attention must be paid to the proportions of minerals to ascorbate that are obtained. A mineral ascorbate molecule contains approximately one part of the mineral to nine parts ascorbic acid. A 500mg tablet of calcium ascorbate, then would contain 50mg of calcium and 450mg of vitamin C. To get 10,000mg of vitamin C daily, 11,500mg of the ascorbate would have to be taken.

Among its everyday functions, ascorbic acid is essential in the synthesis of protein, the formation and maintenance of collagen and other connective tissues, and the assimilation of calcium, iron, and other minerals. It strengthens the spinal discs, helps regulate cholesterol levels, and is involved in the formation of some enzymes and hormones.

Ascorbic Acid concentrates in the optic lens, where it helps maintain normal vision; it is used by antibodies to destroy dangerous bacteria and viruses; and combines with toxins and wastes in the body, neutralizing them and rendering them soluble for excretion. It prevents fatigue by reducing acetone bodies left over when fats are burned for energy. It increases the efficiency of other nutrients, stimulates the growth of healthy intestinal bacteria, and promotes their synthesis of B vitamins.

It is a very effective antioxidant and free-radical deactivator, and reactivates vitamin E that has been oxidized during peroxide deactivation. It also increases the production of lymphocytes, the defense cells of the immune system. Among its special functions, it combats both organic and inorganic poisons, these include mercury, cadmium, lead, arsenic, chromium, and benzene; poison oak and poison ivy; snake, spider, and insect poisons; viral and bacterial toxins (including tetanus and botulism); and many industrial contaminants and pollutants.

It offers significant protection against radiation. It helps to protect against numerous diseases and disorders, including arthritis, rheumatism, poliomyelitis, herpes, mononucleosis, rabies, smallpox, tuberculosis, whooping cough, pneumonia, leprosy, typhoid, typhus, dysentery, cancer, leukemia, atherosclerosis, many forms of heart disease, influenza, and, of course, the common cold.

Other research reports the inclusion of ascorbic acid with inorganic iron, reduces the iron to the ferrous state and enhances its intestinal absorption through maintaining a lower pH for a longer period of time. Ascorbic acid increases the absorption of both ferrous and ferric iron.

Simplifying intake of Supplements

For a number of people, swallowing tablets is a problem. This is particularly so when a therapeutic nutrition and diet is planned which requires supplements be taken three times a day with meals.

a. Psychologically, taking pills is synonymous with taking drugs.

b. Many people have difficulty swallowing pills.

c. For others, the supplements remain undigested due to lack of HCL (hydrochloric acid).

One solution is to place pulverized non-liquid pills and capsules (open capsule and shake out the powder) together and blend. To obtain a correct measurement, the first time this is done do a one day supply and measure the equivalent teaspoon measurement. Then pulverize a weekly supply or a full months supply. Store in a labeled opaque glass bottle. Take the nutrient blend at meal times.

Insufficient stomach acid is particularly problematic for the elderly to digest their food. A glass of organic raw whole milk or apple juice should be taken so that the lactates or malates will keep the digested nutrients ionized as they pass through the alkali duodenum, thereby allowing for greater absorption.

It is most important that these are sipped slowly and used to wash down the blend.

The consumption of fruit and vegetables with meals provides anions which enhance absorption of nutrients.

Medications and Drugs

All medications interfere with the electrolyte chemistry. Extensive research has documented drug-induced deficiency diseases. An excellent book *Drug Induced Deficiency Diseases* written by Professor Daphne Roe presents some insight to the problem.

In another category it is reported that over 500 million dollars are spent annually on antacids to relieve Aacid indigestion. These antacids are effective in alkalizing the acids produced by unnatural food and incorrect food combination. Most users are not aware that there are two kinds of acids:

1. The body has a natural response mechanism when food arrives in the stomach which is to release hydrochloric acid (HCL). This indispensable acid is released in the digestive system and is needed

to digest protein and assimilate certain minerals.

2. As described above, the unnatural acids are caused by unnatural eating and drinking habits.

The problem is that these ant-acids dilute or suppress the essential HCL. HCL is critical to pH during digestion and important to enzyme activity. Medications containing baking soda or bicarbonate of soda are particularly troublesome in disturbing pH.
Baking soda and baking powder, which has baking soda in it, can neutralize the hydrochloric acid in the stomach thus causing indigestion and heartburn and may lead to even more serious gastro-intestinal problems. These highly alkaline substances can also destroy a certain amount of the B-complex in the stomach.

Chapter 9
Toxic Dentistry

Readers of a book about minerals will be surprised to find a chapter about toxic dentistry. The author has unusual research experience with thousands of patients over a number of years linking toxic dentistry to acid pH traced to toxic dentistry.

A vast amount of evidence describes the toxic nature of mercury amalgam fillings. What is not commonly known is that mercury is released as a vapor to absorb into the body tissue causing serious disruption of the electrolyte chemistry resulting in a long list of illness, disease and death!

Whereas researchers have identified the link between mercury and these health problems, they have not understood the link to the disruption of the electrolyte chemistry as the real cause of the problem.

In another category, the mouth is a source of infection and resulting toxicity emanating from the site of root canals and cavitations that are a serious challenge to the immune system and the balance of cellular chemistry.

It seems appropriate as an introduction to this

important chapter to present here a copy of an article that appeared in the ALIVE magazine, the largest circulation of health magazines published in Canada with more than 200,000 readers.

Disease has its Origin in the Mouth!

The evidence is overwhelming. When we submit to common dental procedures, as routinely performed in mainstream dentistry, we submit to a self-inflicted source of toxic poisoning and infection that has no equal in terms of the numbers and variety of resulting illness and disease, suffering and death.

When presented with the devastating diagnosis of a disease such as Multiple Sclerosis (MS), Lou Gehrig's (amyotrophic lateral sclerosis or ALS), Parkinson's or cancer, the patient inevitably responds with the questions. "But doctor--why me? What caused this terrible disease?"

In mainstream medicine the origin of degenerative disease remains a mystery--a situation that will continue as long as there is a focus on treating the symptom and not the cause.

My research has focussed on the need to reveal the origin of all illness and disease. Advanced technology, research and experience working with thousands of patients all provide extensive evidence.

To determine the origin of illness and disease it is essential to reveal imbalances in all systems of the body and then beyond to reveal the causes of these imbalances. Typically this reveals a long list of causal factors. These may include parasites, fungi and bacteria, viruses, toxic metals and chemicals, nutritional deficiencies, pH imbalances and congested energy pathways B to name a few! Once the causal factors are determined, one must delve even further, to the cellular level, to determine their origin.

The shocking truth is that an astonishing number of these evaluations will reveal that the origin of these causal factors is in the mouth!

Amalgam Fillings

Recent studies estimate annual mercury usage by North American dentists ranges from approximately 10,000kg in the 1970's to 170,000kg today. Mercury fillings continue to remain the material preferred by 92 per cent of North American dentists. (The current estimates report that one million amalgams a day are used in the United States alone!)

Although my research of the scientific literature during previous years had revealed extensive evidence linking illness and disease to the infection and toxic metal poisoning of the mouth, the high percentage of patients with disease being traced to the mouth prompted me to return to the scientific literature for a more intensive study of this subject.

A recent landmark study is entitled "Mercury Exposure from 'Silver' Tooth Fillings: Emerging Evidence questions a Traditional Dental Paradigm." It documents the results of research into the pathophysiological effects of amalgam mercury.

This research focuses on the immune system, renal system, oral and intestinal bacteria, reproductive system, and the central nervous system. Other research -- going back 60 years -- presents even more extensive evidence of the toxic side effects in many other systems.

This study confirms that mercury is continuously released as vapor into the mouth; it is inhaled, absorbed into body tissues, oxidized into ionic mercury and produces covalently bound (the sharing of electrons between two atoms, which bonds the atoms) cell proteins. The evidence emphasizes that the toxic effects of amalgam silver fillings have been reported for more than 100 years!

In spite of this long-standing evidence, organized dentistry has countered the controversy surrounding the use of mercury fillings by claiming that mercury reacts with the amalgam metals to form a "biologically inactive substance"--and by stating that dentists have not reported any adverse side effects in patients. Long-term use and popularity continues to be offered as evidence of amalgam safety.

My own experience with patients and their serious conditions are continually traced to toxic metals and, in particular, to infection in the mouth. The resulting diseases include cancer of the breast, brain tumors, throat, nasal, tongue, mouth and skin diseases, MS, ALS, Parkinson's, birth defects and immune deficiency-related illness.

Tooth Decay, Root Canals and Cavitations

Evidence relating to root canals, first published in medical and scientific literature over 60 years ago, is even more substantial. The most well known is the classic research of Dr. Weston Price. Other extensive research, not so well known, was conducted by Patrick Störtebecker, MD, Ph.D.

About 50 years ago, during neurosurgical work on the metastasis of primary tumors throughout the body to the brain, Störtebecker became interested in the valveless cranio-vertebral venous system as a pathway for metastases. His research led him to discover what he described as the "Principle of Shortest Pathway"--the culmination of 30 years of studies presenting evidence of "dental infectious foci and diseases of the nervous system," particularly the spread of microorganisms and their toxins from a peri-apical osteitis (situated at or surrounding the apex of a tooth - inflammation of the bone) within the jaw along the direct cranial venous pathways, eliciting a toxic-infectious encephalopathy.

His well-documented studies include case studies which link root canal infections to MS, encephalitis, epilepsy, schizophrenia, Alzheimer's and Parkinson's diseases, eye diseases and jaw, mouth, throat and brain cancer.

The discovery that the cranial venous system could be filled from the pulp of a tooth initiated further investigation of chronic dental infections in the etiology of glioblastomas (astrocytoma - primary brain tumor and also found throughout the central nervous system).

Störtebecker describes the development of infection invading the jaw bone as peri-apical osteitis and explains how this spreads infection, partly through the cranial venous pathways and partly along the route of trigeminal nerves.

Other research documents a variety of conditions that can have direct links to infected root canals. The number of conditions makes a list too long to publish! They include kidney, liver and gallbladder problems, back, neck and shoulder pain, eye, ear, and skin conditions, neuritis, neuralgia, appendicitis, pneumonia, rheumatism, shingles, arthritis, stomach ulcers, ovarian cysts, testicle infections, intestinal problems, and even hyperactivity in children (the same condition we now refer to as attention-deficit disorder).

Cancer Pathways

It may shock readers that a number of breast cancers have been corrected simply by removing an infected root canal!

To understand this we need to recognize that every tooth in the mouth has an acupressure point connected to a network of more than 800 other acupressure points around which energy flows throughout the body.

In the search for this cancer's origin of pathology, researchers have revealed a pathway from certain molars to the mammary gland. When an infection develops in these teeth, it sets up an inflammatory pathway that will lead to the development of tumors in the breast. When we remove the infected root canal the inflammatory pathway evaporates and the tumors break down or become benign.

This emphasizes the futility of the mainstream approach which focuses on treating the site rather than finding the cause. Similar to the way that oncologists believe that chemotherapy, radiation and surgery are the cure for cancer, so dentists are brainwashed to believe amalgam fillings and root canals are the way to treat dental infections of the teeth. Those who are enlightened are so intimidated by the Canadian and American medical and dental associations, that they knowingly perpetuate treatment, causing suffering and death in the name of medical and dental health rather than providing alternative non-toxic biological dentistry.

In several other countries, there is a move away from toxic dentistry to bio-compatible dental procedures and non-toxic natural dental fillings. A similar move by dentists in the United States and Canada is being aggressively opposed. For information about a biological dentist in your area call the Health Action Network or local naturopathic association.

Pathology Connection to the Mouth

There is an extremely important warning in research regarding the mounting evidence of the damage resulting from problems in the mouth, particularly from amalgam fillings and root canals.

Evidence emphasizes the connection between the release of mercury vapor and cancer of the mouth, brain tumors and not surprisingly, a contributing factor to many degenerative changes in the biochemistry, bioenergetic and biological systems. Amalgams not only release vapor, they block vital energy flow through acupressure points in each tooth.

Root canals become active sites for destructive microbial activity that affect vital systems. Many patients recover following the replacement of mercury amalgams and the removal of root canals.

Another Landmark Study

Note: the author has included as an appendix at the end of this book an abstract from an extensive study published in the scientific literature to demonstrate the evidence against amalgam fillings. This article has technical symbols but important for its historical background especially for cancer patients with several fillings, faced with the opposition to their removal. Hg is the chemical symbol for mercury. In another dimension, this abstract is purposely presented for those medical doctors and dentists confronted with doubts about the connection with cancer.

Chapter 10
Solutions to the Catastrophe

It is incredible, faced with the evidence that our depleted soils are a major factor responsible for the escalating morbidity statistics predicting that one in every third persons is a risk for cancer during their life time, that those at government level responsible for the health of our nation are not taking action to remedy a worsening catastrophe that is causing more deaths than those killed in all of our major wars. Considering the cost of a war and the estimated $750 million spent annually on so called health care, money spent on remineralizing our soils will save billions of taxpayers money, save millions of lives and suffering of millions more Americans.

Four solutions to the Mineral Catastrophe
1. Humic Shale Deposits
2. Cultivation of Fumic Acid
3. Sea Minerals
4. Small grower composting to produce organic grown food.

Humic Shale

There are vast deposits of humic shale that should be used in place of chemical phosphates (NKP) One such site located in Emery, Utah, USA, Rockland Mine claims to be the largest humic shale mine in the world. At the present time, Rockland has more than 1,000 acres of mining leases containing an estimated 320 million metric tons of humic shale reserves (They report this to be sufficient to produce 950 billion gallons of colloidal minerals. The mine reserves could produce enough product to last approximately 500 years if every person in the world drank two ounces of colloidal minerals every day).

However, the use of this humic shale as a replacement for phosphate chemical fertilizer is an obvious solution to the worsening catastrophe of depleted soils; this is especially so as the information gathered insists that the costs of such application would be the same as the chemical fertilizers!

What is Humic Shale?

Humic shale ore is the result of Mother Nature's own incubation. 70 million years ago, Earth's fertile, mineral-rich soil produced wholesome, succulent wild fruit and vegetables and lush green forests. This was an era when, supposedly, the soil near the earth's crust contained at least 84 minerals. The numerous mineral elements available at the time may explain why a tree grew 10 feet in height in its first year, or why the plant-eating brontosaurus reached a body weight of 70,000 pounds yet had a mouth no larger than a horse. According to scientific evidence, all life at that time, whether plant or animal was extremely healthy and assumed that this was a direct result of the plants' ability to extract at least 77 minerals from the soil. (This is a far cry from the number of minerals available from the average soil throughout the world today.)

As the thick growth of vegetation died, it accumulated in large piles and, years later; it was buried from rock and mudflows and deposits of sand and silt. The weight of the overflow compacted or compressed out all of the moisture, and what remains today is a deposit of dried, prehistoric plant derivatives. This is known as humic shale.

Humic shale contains plant derived hydrophilic (water soluble) minerals which are very small in size compared to metallic minerals from ground up rocks and soil. Because plant minerals were, in essence, chelated, digested or pre-assimilated by the plant, they are much more effectively absorbed in a shorter period of time than metallic minerals. The "quicker response" is the direct result of the fact that a plant mineral is predigested which eliminates the time required for total absorption. The additional effectiveness also comes from a hydrophilic mineral's greater overall surface area due to its small size (many small ionic molecules, in an area compared to fewer large molecules).

Many people in the nutrition and agronomy fields predict humic shale ore will eventually change the farming and eating habits of the world. Slowly but surely, humic shale is being recognized as an excellent soil builder to replace minerals in mineral deficient soil. It is easy to understand why this product should be used as a fertilizer or soil enhancer. The average farmer fertilizes mineral deficient soil with only about 4 (mostly metallic) minerals. He could not make a profit if he attempted to fertilize with 10 or 12 minerals. The costs would be prohibitive! However, humic shale contains at least 84 minerals and when comparing the cost to the average metallic industrial fertilizers, is proportionately the same. The humic shale from The Rockland Mine has an extremely high humic acid content that adds to its superior quality.

Additionally, a properly proportioned amount of humic shale in fowl or animal feed is known to provide many benefits overall. This is also easily understood when one realizes the average food (fruit, vegetable, plant or grain) of today only contains about 20 or fewer minerals.

Humic shale can also be utilized for the production of liquid hydrophilic minerals for human and animal consumption. This can be accomplished by placing humic shale in a food grade vat or tank. The shale is then covered with cool, contaminant-free water for a period of days. More than 70 water-soluble minerals are leached from the humic shale to become part of the liquid during this undisturbed leaching period. The leaching time required is dependent upon the mineral strength or total dissolved solids (TDS) desired in the finished product.

The finished product is dark gold in color but brilliantly clear. Hydrophilic minerals never settle out of the liquid. Due to a plant derived hydrophilic mineral's size to weight ratio, it always remains suspended in water in earth's gravitational field. The shelf life of this pure food is indefinite and may be stable for hundreds of years. It will always remain consistent so long as the water is not allowed to evaporate. If evaporation were to occur, powdered minerals would remain. Water added to the powder, becomes a liquid mineral again, with all of the powder in suspension.

After this prehistoric humic shale deposit was discovered in 1926, many trial and error tests revealed that minerals could be extracted from the humic shale with water through a natural leaching process. These plant-derived minerals are being used by increasing numbers of informed individuals.

Nothing such as citric acid or hot water is used to force mineral extraction and nothing is added to the product, not even color. It is one of the purest and most natural products on earth. Each quart of Colloidal Minerals contains approximately 38,000 milligrams of 7 major minerals and approximately 70 trace minerals. As noted earlier, this vast number of minerals seems out of proportion when compared to our fruit, vegetables and grains of today containing an average of 16 to 20 minerals.

Even our meat and dairy products lack the minerals they contained a few short generations ago. Colloidal Minerals can help supplement a body's daily mineral needs, and, because its minerals come from plants, it is one of the most absorbable nutrients one can use. The recommended usage for an average adult is 2 ounces per day mixed with a favorite fruit or vegetable juice.

Fulvic Acid

In another dimension scientists are working to develop fulvic acid and humic substance to deliver mineral concentrations of unbelievable potency.

Scientists have discovered that humic and fulvic acids are the missing link in the human food chain, the lack of which is having deadly consequences. They claim that as a result world health hangs in a fragile balance.

Medical and agricultural research continues to point conclusively to evidence that Fulvic acid holds the keys to prevention, healing, and elimination of the world's diseases!

Fulvic acid is nature's perfect medicine. It is by far the world's most complex and diverse substance. Fulvic acid is actually a whole universe within a single molecule. A good analogy would be to compare the medical implications and complexities of fulvic acid to all the sands of the seashore, where all of the world's man-made pharmaceutical drugs combined would not even rate as one single grain of sand!

The DNA of every living or extinct species of organism on Earth, whether plant, animal, or microorganism, has eventually become a highly refined component of fulvic acid.

The original life giving, protective, and healing components from plants (phytochemicals) do not disintegrate during nature's fulvic acid production process (humification), but become highly concentrated as components of fulvic acid. In a sense you might say these substances are somewhat immortal, they are recycled, reused, and impart vitality and even a certain amount of immortality to subsequent generations of living things.

Fulvic acid exhibits remarkably similar beneficial characteristics to the bioactive substances it originated from, yet the biological effect on other organisms is often significantly magnified and enhanced beyond that of the source material.

Many species of plants, particularly microscopic plants, are involved in the fulvic acid production process, known as humification.

Fulvic acid production is, in essence, nature's perfect recycling process, where the end product, fulvic acid, provides a steady and compounding increase in health to subsequent generations of living organisms.

Modern waste disposal and agricultural practices have completely destroyed nature's fulvic acid production and recycling process, resulting in progressively deteriorating health of crops, animals, and humans.

In a more perfect world, fulvic acid can reverse the steady cycle of health deterioration, and start a new cycle of progressive health improvement.

Fulvic acid is a humic substance or extract. It is the end product of nature's Humification process, which is involved in the ultimate breakdown and recycling of all once-living matter, especially plants.

Fulvic acid contains ALL of the phytochemical protective substances, amino acid peptides, nucleic acids, etc., from the original plant matter, highly concentrated, refined, transformed, and enhanced by the actions of innumerable microscopic plants, such as fungi. The humification processes prevents the original phytochemical protective components from completely breaking down and turning back into basic mineral elements. Even small strands of RNA, DNA, and plant photosynthetic materials still remain intact. Many of the original components become complex enzymes, which have seemingly miraculous function.

Because fulvic acid is so highly refined, it consists of extremely complex but small molecules, easily penetrating cells. For this reason it is highly reactive and bioactive, and is the most rare and valuable of all humic substances. Because of fulvic acid's very small size (low molecular weight), it readily penetrates human tissues and cells, and interacts on the cellular level providing innumerable functions. The results are simply phenomenal.

Nature meant for small amounts of fulvic acid to participate at every level and link along the food chain. It contains latent solar energy and remnants of plant photosynthesis. Fulvic acid even bridges the gap between inert minerals and living matter, and it participates in the spark of life.

Fulvic acid is simply nature's most important form of protection and defense for plants, animals, and man. It is tied very closely with immune system functions and has powerful antioxidant qualities. Because fulvic acid is so small and complex, it has been entirely misunderstood and overlooked by most of medicine and science.

Fulvic Acid Defined

The author supports the notion that fulvic acid is the most miraculous discovery capable of saving our soil and all living things on this planet.

Fulvic acids: What are they? Where do they come from? What can they do? Why do we need them?

Though virtually unknown to the layman, there is perhaps no substance more vital to life (with the possible exception of oxygen and water) than the biologically derived compounds known as Humic and Fulvic acids. Fulvic acids enter into all life processes within plants and animals providing many different life-enhancing benefits to the life cycle on this planet.

They act as free-radical scavengers, supply vital electrolytes, enhance and transport nutrients, catalyzes enzyme reactions, increase assimilation, stimulate metabolism, chelate essential major and trace elements making them organic, and demonstrate amazing capacity for electrochemical balance.

Unknown Fulvic

Despite the fact that scientists world wide have published thousands of papers related to fulvic acids and their effect on living matter, they have received limited public exposure because of the inability to produce and commercialize these substances.

How Are They Formed?

Fulvic acid is a derivative of microbial degradation of humic substances. Microorganisms are essential to the process. Each gram of healthy top soil has in excess of four billion microorganisms that participate in production of bio-chemicals essential to healthy plants and animals. If they were to fail, our lives would cease. A better perspective of their importance can be gained by looking at the work they do.

Microorganism activity in preparing one acre of topsoil expends the equivalent energy of 10,000 people doing the same amount of work in the same amount of time.

What Humic Substances Do in the Soil

Scientists claim organic substances stimulate plant cellular growth and division, including auxin type reactions. They enhance plant circulatory systems and promote optimum plant respiration and transportation systems. They decrease plant stress and premature deterioration. They dramatically improve seed germination and promote greater fibrous root growth. They increase the size and numbers of legume root nodules and increase resistance to drought and insect infestation.

High molecular weight humic substances serve as food stock for microorganisms, which in turn break them down into smaller units of high-energy substances called fulvic acid. Humic substances of high molecular weight, including humic acids, alter the physical characteristics of the soil while low molecular weight fulvic acids are involved in biochemical reactions that influence the plant's metabolic process. Both are indispensable.

The Fulvic Miracle

In addition to duplicating many of the positive functions of humic acid, fulvic acid will:

C Stimulate metabolism C Enhances RNA & DNA C Acts as a catalyst in respiration C Increases metabolism of proteins C Increases activity of multiple enzymes C Enhances the permeability of cell membranes C Enhances cell division and cell elongation C Aids chlorophyll synthesis C Increases drought tolerance, and prevents wilting C Increases crop yields C Assists denutrification by microbes C Buffers soil pH C Contributes electrochemical balance as a donor or an acceptor C Synthesizes new minerals C Chemically weathers inorganic substances C Decomposes silica to releases essential mineral nutrients, detoxifies various pollutants (pesticides, herbicides, etc.)

The two major life functions which cannot be duplicated by man are Photosynthesis and Humification.

Who and What are We?

As has been described, biologically we consist of varying amounts of the following major and minor elements: calcium, carbon, chlorine, hydrogen, iron, iodine, magnesium, sulfur, oxygen, phosphorus, potassium, plus traces of aluminum, bromine, cobalt, copper, fluorine, manganese, nickel, silicon, sodium, zinc, and all the additional (as yet) undiscovered trace elements being added to the list as our knowledge increases.

The Cellular System

The elements we are composed of (plus or minus a few billion) are components of approximately 60 trillion cells. An average cell contains about 1 quadrillion molecules, which is about 10,000 times as many molecules as the milky way has stars. Individual cells when properly nourished, are capable of producing many of their own amino acids, enzymes, and other factors necessary for all metabolic processes. Each cell, in addition to other processes, burns its own energy, maintains itself, manufactures its own enzymes, creates its own proteins, and duplicates itself. It is essential to understand that the total metabolism of the body is the sum of the metabolic operations carried on in each individual cell.

Growth and Maintenance Nutrients

Scientists have identified at least 90 growth and maintenance nutrients which must be continuously supplied to the body to sustain healthful life. These growth and maintenance nutrients include amino acids, major and trace minerals, vitamins and other nutritional factors. When these factors are supplied to our cells, the cells then create the building blocks for the total metabolic machinery of our life process. The building blocks present in the metabolic machinery of human beings are (in the great majority of cases) the same as the building blocks contained in the metabolic machinery of other organisms of extremely different types.

Organisms vary in their capacity to produce some of these building blocks internally. Some organisms are capable of producing all amino acids within their cells. Humans can produce all but eight. Some organisms can produce many of the vitamins within their cells. The very complex processes of all metabolic functions are carried on within the cell.

If we fail to supply the cell with the essential growth and maintenance nutrients we will experience a breakdown of these functions. When this breakdown is substantial we have the onset of disease or the manifestation of some related defect.

Nutritional Deficiencies

Total deficiencies in one or more of the growth and maintenance nutrients which human cells need for healthful metabolism is now a rare occurrence, but substantial deficiencies in the growth and maintenance nutrients is a common factor to every degenerative disease we experience.

Sick Soil, Sick Plants, Sick People

All naturally fertile soils contain adequate amounts of humic and fulvic acids produced by resident microbes within the soil. Humic and fulvic acids assist the plant in obtaining its complete nutrition. Our modern agriculture aims (with few exceptions) at one goal which is to market. Food quality is sacrificed for food quantity. Since the farmer is paid by the bushel, yield is paramount to nutritional content. The farmer in his frantic effort for yield has succumbed to the Pied Pipers of agro-chemical companies with products to sell. He is further decoyed by bad advice from county agents and higher schools of learning that protect the "grant" status of moneys received from these same agro-chemical companies, who advocate the application of excessive amount of nitrate fertilizers to the soil. Such practices stun and destroy the indigenous microbial life within the soil. When microbial life is inhibited or destroyed, vital humic and fulvic acids are exhausted.

Depleting Minerals

When microbes are depleted from the soils, they are no longer present to convert inorganic minerals into organic minerals needed by plants. Excessive use of nitrate fertilizers inhibits the formation of normal plant proteins and stimulates an over-abundance of unused amino acids that attracts insects. Since pests were created to eat diseased plants this introduces the ideal environment for increased infestation because of increased insect food supply. The farmers response is more pesticides and fungicides to save his infested crop. This in turn inhibits or destroys even more vital microorganisms that are essential to mineral conversions to plant nutrients.

Unsafe Food

These deficient, pesticide-laden products are turned into "cash" which the farmer thinks is the bottom line. Lacking in organic trace elements and other nutritional factors, but loaded with chemical residues from pesticides, insecticides, herbicides, these nutritionally depleted products end up on the tables of America. Without taste, and deficient in organic minerals and nutrients, we peel, boil and overcook what remains and ask "why do I hurt?"

Can Good Food Be Found?

A very small percentage of the agricultural lands of America are fertile enough to produce nutritious and healthy food. An honest effort in attempting to select a healthful diet from grocery shelves may be a nutritional disaster. Unless you are fortunate enough to organically grow your own food, supplementation is a necessity.

The Vitamin Connection

In this century common vitamin deficiency diseases have been reduced dramatically due to our awareness of the role of vitamins in nutrition. New breakthroughs are just beginning to emerge in the use of increased dosages for treatment of some ailments. It should be noted however that vitamins cannot complete their function in the cell's metabolism without the presence of certain minerals. This may explain the fascinating effects of humic and fulvic acids at work in living organisms. Fulvic acid chelates and binds scores of minerals into a bio-available form use by cells as needed. These trace minerals serve as catalysts to vitamins within the cell. Additionally, fulvic acid is one of the most efficient transporters of vitamins into the cell.

The Enzyme Connection

An enzyme is a catalyst that does not enter into a reaction but speeds up or causes a reaction to take place. Enzymes are complex proteins. The burning of glucose in cells, for instance, requires the action of several enzymes, each working on the substrate of the previous reaction. Each cell of the body (when properly nourished) is capable of producing the enzymes needed for complete metabolism. Research has shown that fulvic acid improves enzymatic reactions in cells and produces maximum stimulation of enzyme development. The fulvic acid molecule often contains within its structure coenzymes and important factors which the cells may utilize in stimulation of the manufacturing of enzyme reactions and formation. Leading scientists, such as Roger J. Williams, recognize that:

"The building blocks present in the metabolic machinery of human beings are, in the great majority of cases, exactly the same as the building blocks contained in the metabolic machinery of other organism of extremely different types."

Fulvic acid will, in all probability, be found to be one of the key factors of enzyme reactions with all living cells.

Free Radicals and Antioxidants

Free radicals are highly reactive molecules or fragments of molecules that contain one or more unpaired electrons. They circulate through the body causing great mischief in bonding to and injuring the tissues. In addition to destroying tissue, they magnify the probability that injured cells will become susceptible to a great many infections and diseases, or mutate and cause cancer.

Free Radical Scavengers

Most free radicals are oxygen radicals. Our first line of defense against free radicals is a generous supply of free radical scavengers called antioxidants. Dramatic increases of free radicals in our air, food and water in recent years have put a tremendous strain on the body's natural defense mechanisms. When we exceed our capacity to resist, cell membranes and tissues are exposed to the devastating onslaught of free radicals which combine with the lipid portion of cell membranes to greatly lower their resistance to carcinogenic pathogens.

Super Antioxidants

In recent years frantic efforts have been make to locate and isolate compounds with extraordinary affinity for free radicals. Entire industries have evolved around such efforts, with nearly every vendor of health food products offering suitable solutions. Because of the limited public knowledge concerning the great contribution fulvic acid plays as a bidirectional super antioxidant, we need to consider certain facts.

Fulvic Acid and the Free Radical Connection

To gain knowledge of how antioxidants tie up free radicals we need to understand their workings, and explode a general misconception. For antioxidant to bind a free radical, the antioxidant molecule must have unpaired electrons of equal and opposite charge to that one of the unpaired electrons of the free radical. In a sense the free radical scavenger is itself a free radical or it could not mate and neutralize the destructive effects of free radicals.

Fulvic's Unique Multifaceted Capabilities

Scientists have found that fulvic acid is a powerful, natural electrolyte that can act as an acceptor or as a donor in the creation of electrochemical balance. If it encounters free radicals with unpaired positive electrons it supplies an equal and opposite negative charge to neutralize the bad effects of the free radicals. Likewise, if the free radicals carry a negative charge, the fulvic acid molecule can supply positive unpaired electrons to nullify that charge.

Antioxidants and Beyond

Being a bio-available chelated molecule that can "also" chelate, fulvic acid presents another unique capability. As a refiner and transporter of organic minerals and other cell nutrients, it has the ability to turn bad guys into good guys by chelating and humanizing free radicals. Depending upon the chemical makeup of the free radical, they can be incorporated into and become a part of life sustaining bio-available nutrients. They may become an asset instead of a liability. In the event that the chemical makeup of the free radical is of no particular benefit, it is chelated, mobilized, and carried out of the body as a waste product.

The Human Experience

Although being made prior to the discovery and naming of fulvic acid, the late Dr. Clyde Sandgrin publicly stated:

"If I had to chose between the liquid mineral and electricity, electricity would have to go."

Reported benefits are little short of astonishing. For internal use they are:

- Increased energy
- Alleviates anemia
- Chelates body toxins
- Reduces high blood pressure
- Potentizes vitamin and mineral supplements
- Magnifies the effect of herbal teas and tinctures
- Chelates all monovalent and divalent metals
- Is a powerful natural electrolyte
- Restores electrochemical balance
- Stimulates body enzyme systems
- Helps rebuild the immune system

Reported external beneficial use in:

C Treating open wounds C Healing burns with minimum pain or scarring C Eliminating discoloration due to skin bruises C Killing pathogens responsible for athletes foot C Acting as a wide spectrum anti-microbial and fungicide C Treating rashes and skin irritations

C Helping to heal cuts and abrasions C Helping heal insect bites and spider bites C Neutralizing poison ivy and poison oak

Sea Minerals

The sea covers 75% of this planet. The sea abounds with vast resources of unimaginable dimension. Plants demonstrate their mineral contents to be exactly as is in the human body. In fact scientists, including Henry A. Schroeder, M.D., claim that humans originated from the sea. Like the challenge to produce and commercialize fulvic acid, scientists are working to determine how to harvest the rich resources of the sea. Ninety-two elements have been found in the plants that grow in the sea.

An analysis of seawater today shows that it contains about 31 percent sodium, while human blood contains about 34 percent sodium. The concentrations of other elements, such as potassium, calcium, magnesium and chlorine are also overwhelmingly much the same in seawater and blood.

The oceans of the world make up about 75 percent of the earth's surface. They cover about 140 million square miles, with an estimated water volume of approximately 320 million cubic miles. It is inevitable that this vast resource will become an urgent solution to the escalating catastrophe, not only for minerals but also for quality nutrition and healing nutrients for mans many illnesses and disease.

The primary life support system for all mankind is the plant. Plants - from land or sea - are the basis of all life. In the sea, aquatic plants and plankton are the life-giving link. Plankton contains both plant (phytoplankton) and animal (zooplankton) groups. Phytoplankton, by utilizing sunlight and the nutritional treasures of the sea, synthesizes other foodstuffs in water. It begins the food chain for animal life. Many nations harvest both the fish and the vegetation that seas provide, but such use is minimal in the United States. However, times are changing: seaweed is available in Japanese restaurants, and the dried variety is being sold in many markets.

Sea plants

Sea plants have revealed life saving nutrients such as iodine in kelp and dulse. There is no doubt that our vital needs are linked with the sea itself and with sea products. They can: relieve nutritional deficiencies; ease physical discomfort; help produce enzymes within the body itself; contribute to a longer life by helping to guard against small clots within the arteries; improve total health; replace essential minerals and trace minerals; and even provide food alternatives to beef and chicken.

The Japanese are the largest users of seaweed as food. The most commonly eaten seaweed includes Nori, Kombu, Wakame, and Hijiki which is used in the preparation of a soybean paste soup miso.

In another category, often described as the super star of the world's food supply, spirulina, a tiny blue-green algae also referred to as one of nature's original foods, is high in protein, vitamins, minerals and essential fatty acids. It is unique as it is only one cell wide and about a millimeter in length and has an incredible light-sensitive high photosynthesis record of any known land or sea plant. Its other unique properties allow it to recycle carbon dioxide, replacing it with pure oxygen, thus ensuring protection against pollution.

Centuries ago the Aztecs in Mexico harvested the algae, dried in the sun and used as a food staple. People of Chad and Niger harvest the algae from Lake Chad and sell green cakes in the market. Since it is high nutritional quality, easy to produce and economical to market, spirulina has become a commercial crop including supplements in the form of tablets, capsules or powder.

This has led to its cultivation in closed pond conditions. Spirulina can double its mass every few days. Its other unique quality is it is a complete protein supplying all twenty-one amino acids including the essential amino acids which cannot be manufactured in our bodies. Two tablespoons contain approximately thirteen grams of protein. Spirulina can be compared to dried eggs considered the most usable of all protein foods (NPU - net protein utilization - of 94%). Spirulina contains the entire B-complex and the best source of B12 ever to be found. Spirulina has a tough cellulose outer skin that is difficult for some people to digest. This is overcome when HCL is included with the meal.

Composting

Finally, there is the more individualized small grower using composting to produce rich soils growing high quality nutritional vegetables and plant foods. In Alaska, surrounded by mountains and pure glacier water, small farms produce unbelievable vegetables that are entered in seasonal competitions. Incredibly, cabbages grow to 60 pounds in weight, tomatoes the size of watermelons and leeks 3 feet long!

Chapter 11
The Potential of Personal Life Force

It is appropriate to conclude this work with a perception of how the electromagnetic chemistry relates to the life force flowing through the body. In this regard application of the principles explained thus far, lead to a vibrant life force that in itself is a subject of study for those interested in subtle energy healing, and spiritual experience. There is substantial evidence that this life force is interrelated to specific energy centers also described as chakras. Although this book is not intended to be an explanation of these energy systems, drawing attention to this relationship may be the beginning of new dimension for those interested in this subject.

The point here is that when individuals introduce minerals and become aware of a change to more vibrant health many become aware of this vibrant life force. When attention is directed to the subtle energy connection and the potential to transmit this to others, heal others or to develop a new consciousness of a spiritual experience, the impact of minerals and biochemical balance presents a powerful experience that has changed their lives.

Appendices

Appendix A
The Periodic Table

There are 92 natural chemical elements on the Periodic Table. A mineral can be classified as essential if:

It is present in the healthy tissues of the living organism

Its concentration in similar animals and man is fairly constant

Upon withdrawal from the body, reproducible structural and/or physiological abnormalities result

The addition of the deficient mineral corrects the above-mentioned structural and/or physiological abnormalities

An induced deficiency of a specific mineral is always accompanied by a pertinent specific biochemical change
f) The above-mentioned biochemical change can be prevented or corrected when the mineral deficiency is prevented or corrected.

It must be remembered, however, that the mere presence of a mineral such as lead or arsenic in the tissues of the animal or man does not prove it is essential. In fact, it maybe detrimental to the overall health and performance of the organism.

Natural Elements of the Periodic Table in the Universe, excluding the Rare Earths

Understanding the origin and scientific importance of the Periodic Table will clarify the value of the elements described in this book.

Although appearing to be too technical for the average reader, this section is included for future reference when more experience will prompt a return for explanation.

Over a hundred years ago (1871), Dmitri I. Mendeléyeff, a Russian chemist, studied the weights of all the known elements previously discovered on this earth. Knowing something of their properties in solution, he listed them in a specific order of natural occurrence for Mendeléyeff believed in Natural Order of the Universe.

In a sudden flash of inspiration, he detected a periodicity of property and weight. After several trials - in fact many, for the finished product was the result of a number of revisions - he drew up a table of these periodic repetitions, which followed what he called Natural Law.

Because Mendeléyeff was a true genius believing in natural order of the universe, he left blank spaces where he was convinced an element should be, for he was sure that just because an element had not been discovered, there was no reason to think that it could not exist.

To Mendeléyeff came a revelation that was the most important single discovery of modern science, for it opened the fields of chemistry and physics to rational investigation and proved the beautifully simple order of matter in the Universe and the structure of the atom.

Each of Mendeléyeff's blank spaces has since been filled with new elements having properties predicted by him, from atomic numbers 1 through 92, several of them during his lifetime. They were found because he believed that they should be there, or else there was no true order in the Universe.

Furthermore with the burgeoning of the atomic physics, the reasons why the elements fell into a periodic order was discovered in the nature and structure of electrons, (or negative charges), protons (or positive charges), and neutrons (having no charge), which made each atom different.

The radioactive elements, some of which have short lives, fell into place. Their order in terms of weight, structure and chemical properties are shown in the table.

With the stimulus to research resulting from the discovery of fission leading to the atomic bomb, brand new elements were made.

Mendeléyeff had left blank spaces in the actinium series after uranium, No. 92; all have since been filled, from 93 and 94, neptunium and plutonium, to the last, lawrencium, No. 103.

Whether or not man can go further is problematical, for he has to begin a new series, and most of the others have a very short existence, being very unstable - which is why they do not occur naturally.

As this book is concerned with life and living things, we do not need to consider radioactive elements unless they accumulate in living things naturally or from man-made exposures.

All of the elements which are needed by living things are contained in the first 53 of the 92 natural elements on the surface of the earth; all but one occurs in the first 42 and all but two in the first 34.

In the Universe there is a natural order of abundance of the elements, following atomic weight and number. The heavier the element, the less abundant it is.

Furthermore, elements with even atomic numbers are more abundant than elements with odd atomic numbers. This order may not be true now for hydrogen and helium, but it will be eventually in the Sun and Stars. Four hydrogen atoms fuse to make one helium atom, releasing a tremendous amount of energy in the form of light and heat, and one can measure the age of the sun by knowing the proportions of hydrogen and helium. The hydrogen, or fusion bomb, is based on this reaction which is natural in the stars.

No one knows why odd numbered elements are less abundant than even numbered ones. Until we know more of the Master Plan of matter in the Universe we cannot even guess. Nor do we know why the general order of abundance of elements in the Universe according to atomic number is not wholly true on the earth. If it held, lithium and beryllium would be the most abundant solid matter on earth.

All we can guess is that a planet is not wholly representative of the Universe, which we know, and that perhaps these light metals were not formed as readily as heavier ones. But in general, on the earth the order of relative abundance of the elements is the rule, with a number of exceptions, including, of course, the so-called inert gases - which are no longer inert, being made to react with fluorine under special non-universal conditions.

For an element to take part in living matter, it must be:

a) Abundant in sea water b) Reactive; that is, able to join up or bond with other elements c) Able to form an integral part of a structure d) In the case of metals, soluble in water, reactive of itself with

oxygen, and able to bond to organic material - carbon, hydrogen, oxygen, nitrogen, sulfur and phosphorus.

These qualities are found in 23 elements, and perhaps 27, of the first 42 of the Periodic Table.

When looking at the Periodic Table as has been done for many years, one is constantly discovering new bits of information. Look at it horizontally, especially at the elements with numbers 22-30. This is called the first transitional series. Each atom has one or more electrons missing from its outer ring. An atom is like a solar system, the electrons being the planets, which revolve about the central mass of protons of enormous speed. As one goes from titanium, No. 22, to zinc, No. 30, the unfilled orbits change, one electron at a time, changing the properties of each metal in respect to its reactivity. Zinc's outer ring is filled. This transition is similar in Nos. 40-48, and in Nos. 72-80.

Look at the table vertically, each element down from the top row is like the one above, only heavier. Its outer electron ring is exactly like that of the one above, only larger. Therefore, it has the same chemical and physical properties, only a bit different because of size.

Its reactions are the same. It is likely to occur, and does occur, in nature with the one above. Copper, silver and gold occur in the same ores, so do zinc and cadmium, nickel, palladium and platinum, vanadium, niobium and tantalum, chromium, molybdenum and tungsten (wolfram) and so on.

This property is important biologically, especially in terms of reactions and in the possibility of disease. For sizeable amounts of a heavier metal can displace a lighter one in the same group in biological tissues and alter the reaction of the lighter one.

Furthermore, when tissues have an affinity for a certain element or are structured by it, they have an affinity for all other elements of the group. Thus, all Group llA elements are bone seekers, all Group Vll elements are thyroid seekers, all Group llB and VlB are liver and kidney seekers. There seem to be specialized organic compounds in these organs which are avid for certain kinds of elements.

Similar compounds have been manufactured in large varieties by chemists; they are called chelating agents, from the Greek *chela*, a claw. We do not know what these tissue compounds are, but we do find groups of metals in special tissues, particularly when exposures to the abnormal or unnatural elements are heavy.

Further clarification follows:

G	Gas. The inert gases, which are only relatively inert, are shown to the right of the Table. In their molecular, or uncombined states, fluorine and chlorine are gases, but they always occur naturally as compounds.
M	Metal. Metals in Group 1A are alkali metals, in 11A are alkaline earths. They always occur as compounds in nature, with a few exceptions, such as silver, gold, mercury.
C	Non-Metals occurring as compounds, often with oxygen, Group V11A as simple salts of sodium.
TM	Transitional Metal with unfilled outer electron shell, hence reactive.
R	Radioactive, hence unstable to some degree. Elements numbered 84-92 are radioactive: Potassium, Astatine, Radon, Francium, Radium, Actinium, Thorium, Protactinium, Uranium, the last having little radioactivity in its natural state. Most of them are not listed.

At. #	Symbol/Name	State		Symbol/Name	State
1	H Hydrogen	G	30	Zn Zinc	M
2	He Helium	G	31	Ga Gallium	M
3	Li Lithium	M	32	Ge Germanium	M
4	Be Beryllium	M	33	As Arsenic	C
5	B Boron	C	34	Se Selenium	C
6	C Carbon	C	35	Br Bromine	C
7	N Nitrogen	G	36	K Krypton	G
8	O Oxygen	G	37	Rb Rubidium	M
9	F Fluorine	C	38	Sr Strontium	M
10	N Neon	G	39	Y Yttrium	M
11	Na Sodium	M	40	Zr Zirconium	TM
12	Mg Magnesium	M	41	Nb Niobium	TM
13	Al Aluminum	M	42	Mo Molybdenum	TM
14	Si Silicon	C	43	Te Technetium	TMR
15	P Phosphorus	C	44	Ru Ruthenium	TM
16	S Sulphur	C	45	Rh Rhodium	TM
17	Cl Chlorine	C	46	Pa Palladium	TM
18	Ar Argon	G	47	Ag Silver	TM
19	K Potassium	M	48	Cd Cadmium	M
20	Ca Calcium	M	49	In Indium	M
21	Sc Scandium	M	50	Sn Tin	M
22	Ti Titanium	TM	51	Sb Antimony	M
23	V Vanadium	TM	52	Te Tellurium	C
24	Cr Chromium	TM	53	I Iodine	C
25	Mn Manganese	TM	54	Xe Xenon	G
26	Fe Iron	TM	55	Cs Cesium	M
27	Co Cobalt	TM	56	Ba Barium	M
28	Ni Nickel	TM	71	Lu Lutetium	M
29	Cu Copper	TM	72	Hf Hafnium	TM

Atomic No.	Symbol	State	Atomic No.	Symbol
73	Ta Tantalum	TM	85	AT Astatine
74	W Wolfram (Tungsten)	TM	86	Rn Radon
75	Re Rhenium	TM	87	Fr Francium
76	Os Osmium	TM	88	Ra Radium
77	Ir Iridium	TM	103	Lr Lawrencium
78	Pt Platinum	TM	104	Rf Rutherfordium
79	Au Gold	TM	105	Ha Hahnium
80	Hg Mercury	M	106	Sg Seaborgium
81	Tl Thallium	M	107	Bh Bohrium
82	Pb Lead	M	108	Hs Hassium
83	Bi Bismuth	M	109	Mt Meitnerium
84	Po Polonium	MR	110	Ds Darmstadtium

Lanthinide Series - first in the series, the rare-earth metals. They often occur together naturally. Many forms colored, usually tripositive, ions that are strongly paramagnetic.

Actinide Series - a group of radioactive chemical elements from element 89 (actinium) through element 103 (lawrencium): it resembles the lanthanide series in electronic structure.

Lanthanide Series

Atomic Number	Symbol	Atomic Number	Symbol
57	La Lanthanum	64	Gd Gadolinium
58	Ce Cerium	65	Tb Terbium
59	Pr Praseodymium	66	Dy Dysprosium
60	Nd Neodymium	67	Ho Holmium
61	Pm Promethium	68	Er Erbium
62	Sm Samarium	69	Tm Thulium
63	Eu Europium	70	Yb Ytterbium

Actinide Series

Atomic Number	Symbol	Atomic Number	Symbol
89	Ac Actinium	96	Cm Curium
90	Th Thorium	97	Bk Berkelium
91	Pa Protactinium	98	Cf Californium
92	U Uranium	99	Es Einsteinium
93	Np Neptunium	100	Fm Fermium
94	Pu Plutonium	101	M Mendelevium
95	Am Americium	102	No Nobelium

Appendix B
Mineral Interaction Chart

The late Professor Eric Underwood stated, that a-metabolic interactions among trace elements are so potent and so diverse that no consideration of the current status of nutrition would be reasonable without some account of their nutritional implications. Trace metal interactions are more frequent among elements that share common chemical parameters and compete for common metabolic sites.

All minerals interact with and influence each other, and a balance between them must be maintained if health and nutrient efficiency are to be achieved. Those minerals that are involved in many metabolic processes are more likely to be interrelated, one to another, than those involved in a single function.

One of the first valid studies on mineral interactions was published in 1954 by Dick, A., *Studies on the Assimilation and Storage of Copper in Sheep*. He reported that there was a three-way interaction between copper, molybdenum and sulfur as a sulfate. Since that first study, other mineral relationships have been investigated and established as valid interactions.

Similar studies were being conducted in plants at about the same period of time. In 1953, D. Mulder (in *Les Elements Mineurs en Culture Furitiere*) first showed the complexity of mineral reactions even in plants with his Interaction Chart. This is seen in this figure.

Using this mineral interaction concept for only one application, that of intestinal absorption of ions from ingested soluble inorganic mineral salts that are competing for carrier molecules and/or intestinal absorption sites, I. Dyer (*Mineral Requirements*) expanded Mulder's interaction Chart and applied it to animals. Even so, he only showed the antagonism between the various mineral nutrients when ingested as salts. This is seen in the next figure. The arrows indicate antagonism between minerals as they compete for absorption sites and/or carrier molecules.

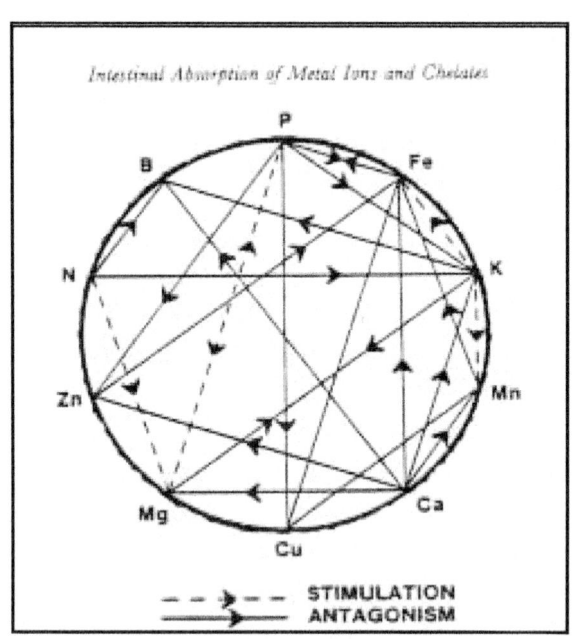

N. Suttle, (*Trace Element Interactions in Animals*), has grouped these minerals interactions show in Figure 2 into six categories according to the type of mechanism involved in causing the interaction which in turn influences absorption of each mineral.

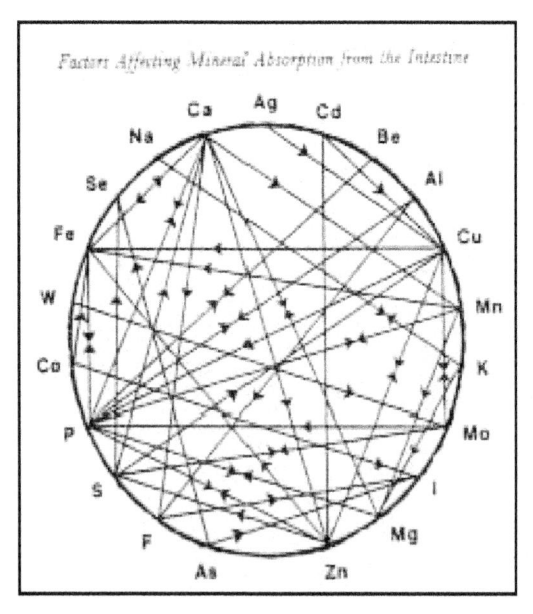

Factors Affecting Mineral Absorption from the Intestine

The first category involves the formation of insoluble complexes. The primary action often involves only one mineral plus a precipitating ligand. The interaction occurs when minerals compete for the same anionic ligand. The ligand may be inorganic, such as a phosphate, or organic such as a phytate.

The complexing with a precipitating ligand can occur in the tissues wherein a mineral can displace another mineral from its position in the tissue. The displaced mineral is then free to enter into a reaction with a precipitating ligand.

More appropriate to this discussion are the interactions occurring in either diet and/or the digestive tract. Again there is competition among the minerals for the precipitating ligand. The competition depends upon the concentrations of the minerals involved, the relative strengths of the association constants of the minerals, and the solubility of the product.

Precipitating substances derived from the diet are a major factor affecting intestinal absorption of metal. Once the mineral salt is ionized in preparation for membrane transport of the cation, it is by its very physical nature unstable. In the ionic state it is highly susceptible to sequencing by phytic acid from cereals and other plant seeds. The phytic acid forms very stable complexes with mineral ions rendering them unavailable for intestinal uptake because the first step in mineral absorption requires that the mineral remain in the ionic state. As the phytic acid content of the diet

increases, the intestinal absorption of certain metals, specifically zinc and calcium and presumably others, decreases. The reduction in mineral phytate absorption may be due to the lack of ionization of the mineral complex in the stable phytate form. If precipitation were to occur, there would be no inducement for carrier proteins located on the intestinal cell membrane to bind themselves to the metal ion prior to membrane transport because the metal is not in ionic form.

The same general principal holds true for other mineral precipitating substances found in the diet such as oxalates, and probably more importantly from a dietary point of view, phosphates. Calcium, magnesium, zinc, iron, aluminum and beryllium all react with dietary phosphates to form insoluble precipitates. Most phosphates are slightly soluble in water or acid solutions. However, the intestine tends to become alkaline which reduces the solubility of the phosphates when introduced into that environment. When the mineral is trapped within an insoluble compound, there is little likelihood of significant intestinal absorption since the precipitated salt is generally stable, creating no attraction to induce integral carrier proteins in their lipid environment in the membranes of mucosal cells to bind the ion and move across the membrane.

The second group of mechanisms that influences

intestinal absorption of minerals involves the competition of chemically similar ions for the same transport carriers. The gut is an important site for these interactions. For example, carrier proteins of small molecular weight can be found in the duodenum. These carrier proteins are subject to competition among the ions for their binding and consequential absorption. The competition can be between micro- and macro-minerals.

The investigations of El-Shobaki and Rummel illustrate this interaction. They found that copper is preferentially bound to transferrin, the protein transport molecule in the mucosa, when competing with iron. Normally, this transport mechanism is not completely saturated, so there are adequate binding sites for both the iron and the copper. Nevertheless, when copper and iron are administered to an excess, iron absorption is inhibited because of the preferential binding of copper to the transferrin. This displacement is based on the ability of the organic molecule to change the electromotive potential of the iron. In other words, some metals will be bound to the carrier protein before others, and a displacement can occur if a stronger metal requires the binding site held by the weaker metal.

The third mechanism that may affect mineral uptake is not directly related to intestinal absorption; although there is some evidence that a similar mechanism may possibly exist in the gut. It involves the synthesizing of metal-binding proteins by the body as a specific reaction to heavy metal loading. The proteins are not specific for the toxic mineral per se, and they may bind other minerals, thus participating in trace mineral interactions. The full significance of these metalloproteins is yet to be elucidated.

A change in the metal component of a metalloenzyme is the fourth mechanism involved in mineral absorption. As previously alluded to, a metal that activates a specific enzyme can be replaced by another metal that may either block or accelerate that particular enzymatic activity. For example, the carboxypeptidase enzyme is activated by zinc. The zinc can be replaced by cobalt, which will cause a decrease in peptidase activity.

Most mineral competition obviously occurs in the plasma and tissues instead of the gut, because the majority of the enzymatic activity within the body occurs in the tissues and plasma. Nevertheless, digestive enzyme activity does influence mineral absorption. The competition of different minerals for those enzymes therefore influences their overall absorption.

The fifth mechanism involving mineral interactions is related to the second mechanism, that of metabolic pathways. More specifically, it involves the transport and excretion of the minerals. Some of these transport mechanisms are in the intestinal cell membrane, while others are in the mucosal cells themselves. From available data from the plasma and extrapolated to the mucosa it appears that only specific interrelationships are involved as they relate to specific transport mechanisms.

The last mechanism has the least significance to mineral nutrition, but nevertheless is important in the overall view of mineral interactions. In each of the above, the mineral interaction has been considered separately, but many interactions are precipitated and/ or affected by other interactions occurring concurrently. To illustrate, the precipitating of a mineral with an insoluble ligand will interfere with the ability of that specific metal to enter into other enzymatic interactions which in turn can affect the uptake of still other minerals which were not affected by the precipitating ligands directly.

Not only do minerals interfere with the absorption of other minerals, but other nutrients, such as vitamins, can have equally significant positive or negative influence on mineral absorption. Vitamin D is one such example. Its role is in the regulation of intestinal absorption of ionic calcium has been conclusively proven.

Appendix C
Mercury Exposure from Silver Tooth Fillings

Emerging Evidence Questions a Traditional Dental Paradigm

For more than 160 years, dentistry has used silver amalgam, which contains approximately 50% Hg (chemical symbol for the element mercury) metal as the preferred tooth filling material. During the past decade medical research has demonstrated that this Hg is continuously released as vapor into mouth air; then it is inhaled, absorbed into body tissues, oxidized to ionic Hg, and finally covalently bound to cell proteins.

Animal and human experiments demonstrate that the uptake, tissue distribution, and excretion of amalgam Hg is significant, and that dental amalgam is the major contributing source to Hg body burden in humans.

Current research on the pathophysiological effects of amalgam Hg has focussed upon the immune system, renal system, oral and intestinal bacteria, reproductive system, and the central nervous system. Research evidence does not support the notion of amalgam safety.- Lorscheider, F.L., Vimy, M.J., Summers, A.O.

Mercury exposure from "silver" tooth fillings: emerging evidence questions a traditional dental paradigm. Faseb j. 504-508 (1995). Key words: Mercury Toxicity. Dental Amalgam.

Historical Overview of Mercury use in Dentistry

As early as the 7th century, the Chinese used a "silver paste" containing mercury (Hg) to fill decayed teeth. Throughout the Middle Ages, Alchemists in China and Europe observed that this mysterious silvery liquid, extracted from cinnabar ore, was volatile and would quickly disappear as a vapor when mildly heated.

Alchemists were fascinated that at room temperature Hg appeared to "dissolve" powders of other metals such as silver, tin, and copper.

By the 1800s, the use of a Hg/silver paste as a tooth filling material was being popularized in England and France and it was eventually introduced into North America in the 1830s. Some early dental practitioners expressed concerns that the Hg/silver mixture (amalgam) expanded after setting, frequently fracturing the tooth or protruding above the cavity preparation, and thereby prevented proper jaw closure.

Other dentists were concerned about mercurial poisoning; because it was already widely recognized that Hg exposure resulted in many overt side effects, including dementia and loss of motor coordination. By 1845, as a reflection of these concerns, the American Society of Dental Surgeons and several affiliated regional dental societies adopted a resolution that members sign a pledge not to use amalgam.

Consequently, during the next decade some members of the society were suspended for the malpractice of using amalgam. But the advocates of amalgam eventually prevailed and membership in the American Society declined, forcing it to disband in 1856. In its place arose the American Dental Association, founded in 1859, based on the advocacy of amalgam as a safe and desirable tooth filling material. Shortly thereafter, tin was added to the Hg/Silver paste to counteract the expansion properties of the previous amalgam formula.

There were compelling economic reasons for promoting dental amalgam as a replacement for the other common filling materials of the day such as cement, lead gold, and tinfoil. Amalgam's introduction meant that dental care would now be within the financial means of a much wider sector of the population, and, because amalgam was simple and easy to use, dentists could readily be trained to treat the anticipated large number of new patients.

By 1895, the dental amalgam mixture of metals had been modified further to control for expansion and contraction, and the basic formula has remained essentially unchanged since then. Scientific concerns about amalgam safety initially surfaced in Germany during the 1920's, but eventually subsided without a clear resolution.

At the present time, based on 1992 dental manufacturer specifications, amalgam (at mixing) typically contains approximately 50% metallic Hg, 35% silver, 9% tin, 6% copper, and a trace of zinc. Estimates of annual Hg usage by the U.S. dentists range from approximately 100,000 kg in the 1970s to 170,000 kg today. Hg fillings continue to remain the material preferred by 92% of U.S. dentists.

Presently, organized dentistry has countered the controversy surrounding the use of Hg fillings by claiming that Hg reacts with the amalgam metals to form a "biologically inactive substance" and by observing that dentists have not reported any adverse side effects in patients. Long-term use and popularity also continues to be offered as evidence of amalgam safety.

In light of the medical research evidence that has accumulated primarily over the past decade, the purpose of this review is to examine the traditional dental paradigm that maintains that amalgam is a biologically safe and appropriate tooth restorative material.

Mercury Exposure from Amalgam Fillings

During the early 1980s several laboratories established that Hg vapor (Hg^0) is continuously released from amalgam tooth fillings, and that the rate released into human mouth air is increased immediately after chewing or tooth brushing. Mouth air levels of Hg correlate significantly with the number of occlusal (biting) amalgam surfaces in molar teeth. Continuous chewing for 10-30 minutes results in a sustained elevation of the mouth Hg0 level, which eventually declines to a baseline level 90 minutes after chewing cessation. Blood Hg levels also display a positive correlation with the number and total surface area of amalgam fillings.

A single amalgam filling with an average surface area of only 0.4 cm^2 is estimated to release as much as 15 Fg (micrograms) of Hg/day primarily through mechanical wear and evaporation, but also through dissolution into saliva. Recent electron microscopy images and electrochemistry data show direct evidence of amalgam Hg corrosion and leakage into saliva as free ions. Thus for an average individual with eight occlusal amalgam fillings, a total of 120 Fg Hg could be released daily into the mouth and a portion of this amount would be inhaled or swallowed.

These estimates are consistent with a recent report showing that human subjects with an average number of amalgam fillings excrete approximately 60 Fg Hg/day in feces, a portion of which is micro-particles of amalgam. Various laboratories have estimated that the average daily body adsorption of amalgam Hg in humans ranges between 1.2 and 27 Fg, with levels for some individual subjects being as high as 100 Fg/day.

At the present time the consensus average estimate is 10 Fg of amalgam Hg absorbed per day, an uptake amount corroborated by a more recent daily of 12 Fg. By way of contrast, estimates of the daily adsorption of all forms of Hg from fish and seafood is 2.3 Fg, and from other foods, air, and water is 0.3 Fg.

Thus, it is now proposed that dental amalgam tooth fillings are the major source of Hg exposure of the general population. This position has been clearly validated by a recent demonstration that at least 65% of excretable Hg in human urine is derived solely from dental amalgams, and that amounts of Hg excreted also correlate with total amalgam surface area.

Body Tissue Uptake of Amalgam Mercury

The degree to which body tissues can sequester amalgam Hg after exposure has been demonstrated in a variety of human and animal experiments. Human autopsy studies reveal significantly higher Hg concentrations in brain and kidney of subjects with aged amalgam fillings than in subjects who had no amalgam tooth restorations. When amalgam fillings containing a radioactive Hg tracer were placed in sheep molar teeth, a whole-body image scan performed 4 weeks later demonstrated several possible uptake sites for Hg including oral tissues, jaw bone, lung, and gastrointestinal tract, with major localization of Hg in the kidney and liver.

A similar whole-body image study repeated in a monkey (whose teeth, diet feeding regimen, and chewing pattern more closely resemble those of humans) clearly demonstrates high levels of amalgam Hg in kidney, intestinal tract, and other tissues. The brain - CSF (cerebrospinal fluid) Hg ratio had increased threefold by 4 weeks after amalgam fillings had been installed. The primate kidney will continue to accumulate amalgam Hg for at least 1 year after installation of such fillings.

Repeated observations in adult sheep demonstrate that after placement of amalgam fillings, the blood Hg levels remain relatively low even though the surrounding body tissue concentrations of Hg become many fold higher than blood. This suggests that tissues rapidly sequester amalgam Hg at a rate equivalent to its initial appearance in the circulation.

Such a phenomenon may explain why monitoring blood levels of Hg in humans is a poor indicator of the actual tissue body burden directly attributable to continuous low-dose Hg exposure from amalgam.

In pregnant sheep, which received amalgam fillings containing a radioactive Hg tracer, it was demonstrated that both maternal and fetal tissues began to accumulate amalgam Hg within several days after such filling were installed. Maternal-fetal transfer of amalgam

Hg also transferred to breast milk postpartum. More recently, human fetal/neonatal studies have likewise demonstrated that Hg concentrations in fetal kidney and liver, and cerebral cortex of infants, correlate significantly with the number of amalgam filled teeth of their mothers.

This latter finding is consistent with previous animal studies that show greater Hg concentration in rat fetal tissues (and less placental retention) when the source of exposure was Hg^0 rather than mercury salts.

Cell Metabolism of Mercury - Major Metabolic Pathways

The principal source of Hg^0 is vapor from dental amalgam tooth fillings, whereas organic Hg (Hg^+) is derived principally from fish and seafood, and inorganic Hg (Hg^{2+}) originates from other foods, water and air.

Approximately 80% of inhaled Hg^0 is absorbed across the lung and converted to Hg^{2+} intra-cellularly by catalase oxidation. In contrast to other Hg species, the high lipid solubility of Hg^0 permits it to cross cell membranes readily, including the blood-brain barrier, and easily enter the brain. However, the kidney eventually becomes the major site of Hg accumulation during compartmental redistribution after exposure to Hg^0.

Some Hg^0 is also dissolved in saliva and swallowed, converted to Hg^{2+} by peroxidase oxidation, and the majority is eliminated by fecal excretion. Other Hg^{2+} that is ingested in the diet is poorly absorbed across the intestinal tract and most is excreted in the feces. Although the majority of substantial portion is absorbed intra-cellularly as methyl-Hg^+. Both intracellular

Hg^{2+} and Hg^+ are ultimately bound covalently to glutathione (GSH - reduced glutathione) and protein cysteine groups. Hg^{2+} is the toxic product responsible for the adverse effects of inhaled Hg^0.

Body tissues have various retention half-lives for Hg^+ and Hg^{2+} ranging from days to years. After Hg is released from tissues, fecal excretion becomes the predominant route for elimination of Hg from the body. Human fecal excretion of Hg correlates significantly with the number of amalgam fillings, and the excretion rate for Hg in feces is 20 times higher than its corresponding excretion rate in urine.

Even though fecal excretion of amalgam Hg predominates, this principal excretory route in humans shows a high correlation with urinary excretion of Hg. Fecal excretion rates for Hg in human subjects with amalgam tooth fillings can be as much as 100-fold higher than in subjects without such fillings.

Significance of Glutathione and other Sulfhydryl Compounds

The major low molecular weight sulfhydryl compound in mammals is GSH, present at approximately 5 mm in cells, serum and bile. Other low molecular weight sulfhydryl is present at lower concentrations in cells include cysteine, biotin, lipoic acid, and coenzyme A. The major targets in proteins for binding of transition metals, including Hg, are the sulfhydryl group of cysteine and the amino nitrogen of histidine. The aromatic ring nitrogens of the nucleotide bases also form Hg complexes, with thymine and uracil being more reactive than cytosine, guanine, and adenine.

Whereas Hg^0 from amalgam is lipid soluble and freely passes through cell membranes, methyl and ionic Hg from food and other sources are both charged and therefore must be complexed with counter-ions or low molecular weight sulfur compounds in order to pass freely through the cell membrane.

The major cellular reaction potentiating the toxicity of Hg^0 is its oxidation by catalase, an enzyme found in all normal mammalian cells. This oxidation process can take place in any of the "barrier tissues" of the body as well as in the blood. Once generated within the cell by catalase, highly reactive Hg^{2+} will interact with a variety of nucleophilic ligands, the most abundant single nucleophile reactant being GSH. The sulfhydryl groups of proteins are next in abundance and avidity for Hg^{2+}, with the amino nitrogens of histidine and the nucleobases being substantially less reactive.

Despite the large molar excess of GSH, many proteins compete very effectively for binding of transition metals such as Zn (zinc), Ni (nickel), and Cu (copper). The precise chemical basis for the high affinity of such metalloproteins (a protein that has one or more tightly bound metal ions forming part of its structure) is not understood. Many of the currently well-defined members of this group, including important regulatory proteins, use cysteines and histidines as ligands to their respective metal cofactors. Thus, these proteins may exchange metals, including Hg, bound to GSH.

Once bound to GSH, Hg can leave the cell to circulate in serum or lymph and be deposited in other organs or tissues. GS-Hg-SG is eventually eliminated via either the kidney or down loaded via bile into the intestinal lumen and excreted in feces. After Hg leaves cells, its major route of elimination in any form (inorganic or organic) is via feces, with less than 10% of Hg normally exiting the body in urine.

Experiments in sheep and monkey indicate that 99% amalgam Hg is excreted in feces and in humans with 30 amalgam surfaces the average 24 hour excretion rate for Hg in feces is 60 micrograms (95% of total daily excretable Hg) in contrast to 3 micrograms / 24 hour in urine. In mammals half-lives from acute single doses of Hg^{2+} or methyl-Hg^+ range from months to years. Half-lives may differ with chronic Hg exposure as a result of compromise cellular function (e.g. kidney Hg turn over diseases with age and duration of exposure).

Effects of Amalgam Mercury on Cell and Organ System Function

The overt clinical effects resulting from toxic exposure to the three species of Hg have been described. Various animal and human experiments over the past several years have addressed the possibility of more subtle pathophysiological effects of amalgam Hg upon the function of several organ system of cell types, including the immune system, renal system, oral and intestinal bacteria, reproductive system, and central nervous system.

Immune System

Ionic Hg has been shown to be antigenic and capable of inducing autoimmunity in rats. In a very recent report, gelatin encapsulated dental amalgam pieces were implanted intraperitoneally in an inbred strain of mice known to be genetically susceptible to Hg-induced pathology. Within 10 weeks to 6 months the animals displayed hyperimmunoglobulinemia (a set of related recurrent skin and lung infections), serum autoantibodies that targeted nucleolar proteins, and systemic immune complex deposits.

Similar changes were observed when only dental alloy (not containing Hg) was implanted, in these immune aberrations were attributed to the silver component of the alloy. This study concluded that both Hg and silver dissolution from dental amalgam can chronically stimulate the mouse immune system with subsequent induction of systemic autoimmunity. In humans, fecal excretion of silver is also correlated with the number of amalgam fillings. This would suggest that further investigation of the potential molecular effects of amalgam metals on the human immune system is warranted.

Renal System

Because human, monkey and sheep kidney display significantly increased Hg concentrations after exposure to dental amalgam, some investigations have focussed on what these concentrations may imply for renal function. Sheep with amalgam tooth fillings implants show a reduced filtration rate of inulin, increased urinary excretion of sodium, and a decrease in urinary albumin.

An increased sodium excretion has also been observed in monkeys similarly treated with amalgam fillings (unpublished data). Because Hg^{2+} accumulates primarily in the proximal tubule of rat and rabbit kidney and amalgam Hg in the proximal tubule of monkey kidney, where the majority of sodium is normally reabsorbed, increased excretion of sodium after placement of amalgam fillings in sheep may reflect a reduced tubular capacity to conserve sodium selectively. Urinary albumin levels increased 1 year after removal of amalgam fillings in humans, whereas urine albumin levels fell in sheep after amalgam placement. It is uncertain whether these differences in albumin excretion patterns may reflect a Hg-induced reduction in renal blood flow due to the presence of amalgam fillings.

Oral and Intestinal Bacteria

It is well established that some human intestinal bacteria carry plasmids encoding resistance to both Hg and antibiotics. In a population subgroup of 356 persons who had no recent antibiotic exposure, those individuals with a high prevalence of Hg resistant bacteria in their intestinal flora were significantly more likely to display multiple antibiotic resistance in these same bacteria. A parallel investigation in monkeys demonstrated a marked increase in the proportion of Hg-resistant bacteria in the floras of the intestine and oral cavity soon after installation of dental amalgam tooth filling were removed. The majority of these primate Hg resistant bacteria was also resistant to one or more commonly used antibiotics. Results show that Hg released form dental amalgam can enhance the prevalence of resistance to multiple antibiotics in the bacteria of the primate normal flora.

Reproductive System

The relationship of occupational exposure to Hg^0 and fertility of female dental assistants has recently been examined, because it is well established that long-term exposure to Hg^{2+} will alter reproductive cyclicity in rodents. Epidemiological screening by questionnaire of 7000 dental assistants showed that within an eligible subgroup of 418 women who were subsequently interviewed, fertility was reduced to only 63% that of control women not occupationally exposed to Hg.

The study, while open to the criticism of all data that rely upon subjective observation and opinion, concluded that dental assistants who prepared 30 or more amalgam fillings per week, and who also had poor Hg hygiene habits, were at risk of lowered fertility.

Central Nervous System

Initially suggestions occurred within medicine that neural-degenerative diseases could perhaps be liked to Hg from dental amalgam, but no experimental evidence was available at that time. However, it is now established that uptake and accumulation of amalgam Hg occur in monkey and human brain tissues.

Studies have demonstrated that Hg is selectively concentrated in human brain regions involved with memory function (medial basal nucleus, amygdala, and hippocampus), and have suggested that Hg may be implicated (by mechanisms as yet unexplained) in the etiology of Alzheimer's disease (AD). Abnormal microtubule formation in AD brains has been associated with a defect in the tubulin polymerization cycle, which may increase the density of neurofibrillary tangles.

A similar tubulin defect can be induced in the brain of HgCl2-treated rats, suggesting a connection between exposure to inorganic Hg and AD. HgCl2 also markedly inhibits in vivo ADP-ribosylation of two rat brain cytoskeletal proteins, tubulin and actin, and thus alters a specific neurochemical reaction involved in maintaining brain neuron structure.

It is well established that Hg^+ will interact with tubulin resulting in disassembly of microtubules, and that microtubules function to maintain neurite structure. In a current investigation, recently reported, rats were exposed to Hg^0 4h/day for as long as 14 consecutive days.

Vapor exposure was maintained at 300Fg Hg/m^3 air, a level detectable in mouths of some human subjects with large numbers of amalgam fillings. Average brain Hg concentrations increased significantly with duration of Hg^0 exposure.

Photo-affinity labeling of the B-subunit of the tubulin dimmer with $[a^{32}P]8N3GTP$ in brain homogenates was diminished by 75% after 14 days of Hg^0 exposure. An identical neurochemical lesion of similar magnitude was seen in human AD brain homogenates, but no direct evidence exists to prove that this lesion is the result of human exposure specifically to amalgam Hg.

Because the rate of tubulin polymerization is dependent on binding of tubulin dimmers to GTP, it was concluded that chronic inhalation of low-level Hg^0 in rats can inhibit the polymerization of tubulin essential for formation of microtubules.

Another recent report demonstrates subclinical neuropsychological and motor control effects from an occupational exposure to Hg^0 over 1 year in a sub-population of dentists with high urinary Hg levels. A more extensive report, evaluating dental technicians and dentists who received occupational exposure to Hg^0 and non-chelation drug (DMPS) challenge test urinary Hg levels were 16-fold higher in technicians and 6-fold higher in dentists compared to control subjects.

Baseline urinary porphyrin levels measured before DMPS treatment were associated with urinary Hg levels obtained after the DMPS challenge. Urinary Hg was also adversely associated with several neurobehavioral changes in Hg-exposed subjects including impairment of attention tasks and motor perceptual tasks. The utility of a DMS challenge to assess renal Hg burden was established.

Conclusions

The collective results of numerous research investigations over the past decade clearly demonstrate that the continuous release of Hg^0 from dental amalgam tooth fillings provides the major contribution to Hg body burden. The experimental evidence indicates that amalgam Hg has the potential to induce cell or organ pathophysiology. At the very least, the traditional dental paradigm, that amalgam is a chemically stable tooth restorative material and that the release of Hg from this material is insignificant, is without foundation.

One dental authority states that materials are presently available that are suitable alternatives to Hg fillings. Based on recent immunology investigations, electrochemical corrosion experiments, and human metabolic studies, it appears that the use of silver in amalgam may be almost as questionable as is Hg, and this evidence suggests that it may be inappropriate to alternatively use recently developed Hg-free silver-containing dental metals to fill teeth. It would seem that now is the time for dentistry to use composite (polymeric and ceramic) alternatives and discard the metal alchemy bestowed on its profession from a less enlightened era.

Although human experimental evidence is incomplete at the present time, recent medical research findings presented herein, strongly contradict the unsubstantiated opinions pronounced by various dental associations and related trade organizations, who offer their opinion without providing hard scientific data, including animal, cellular and molecular evidence, to support their claims.

Acknowledgment from the Author

The author thanks the Wallace Genetic Foundation, the International Academy of Oral Medicine and Toxicology, the University of Georgia Research Foundation, and the National Institutes of Health, whose support of research contained in a number of the citations herein made this review possible.

Appendix D
pH Saliva Test

One of the most important developments in research on deficiency disease was the development of a simple yet accurate clinical test for calcium deficiency. When healthy, the pH of the blood is 7.4, the pH of the spinal fluid is 7.4, and the pH of the saliva is 7.4. Thus, the pH of the saliva is comparable to the extracellular fluid. Calcium (mono) orthophosphate is a major component of these chemical buffer body fluids that tries to maintain pH at 7.4. pH is critical in promoting both normal DNA synthesis, cell growth, cell function, and cell repair. As the level of the chemical buffer drops in these serums, so too does the ability to maintain this critical pH.

The calcium ion level therefore has a direct reflection on the pH. This can be measured by a simple three second, two cent, pH test of the saliva that provides an immediate indication of the state of the calcium ion level, and thus indirectly the state of our health.

The pH of the fluids inside the cell drops from the alkaline negative pH of 7.4 when the channels are open, to as low as the acidic positive pH of 6.6 after the channels close and the nutrients have been chemically altered and consumed by the cell. This change in pH creates the potential difference (voltage) between the inside cellular fluids and the outside fluids, resulting in the channels opening again.

This process is repeated indefinitely like a cell breathing process. When discharged into the cell, this electrical potential activates all of the biological processes that are responsible for cell function and nerve stimulus.

If the pH of the extracellular fluids falls to a level lower than 7.4, as an example to a pH 6.5 due to chronic calcium deficiency, then the intracellular fluids must drop lower, to about 6.3 to produce the same electrical voltage difference. This causes the nutrient glucose to stop producing the A, C, G and T radicals required for normal DNA synthesis and instead to produce lactic acid, which drops the pH even further. The result is a weakening of cell function. If the extracellular pH drops even further, the intracellular pH drops correspondingly, and may result in the production of toxic enzymes as well as cellular breakdown. This is reflected as disease, the aging process, and the production of cell mutations.

Mother Nature tries to keep this from readily occurring by providing a second buffer mechanism: a mixture of potassium dihydrogen phosphate and disodium hydrogen phosphate that can maintain the extracellular serum at a pH of 6.8. Unfortunately, in this case, the large potassium ion has great difficulty in leaving the cell once inside; however, this tends to raise the pH slightly. Thus this secondary support buffer system is much more limited in its capability of keeping the pH from dropping.

It is therefore evident that the physical pH test of saliva represents the most consistent and definitive sign of the ionic calcium deficiency syndrome. It has been found acidic pH is directly related to unnatural lifestyle habits that supported the calcium deficiency, and all of the various stages of developing ionic calcium deficiency and disease. When deficiencies are created by defects in lifestyle are corrected by diet and dietary supplements, the pH rises as disease regresses.

The pH paper can be obtained by the general public through most pharmacies. It comes in various ranges, and the range between 4.5 and 7.5 is best. The pH range of the non-deficient and healthy person is in the 7.5 - dark blue, to 7.00 - blue, slightly alkaline range. The range from 6.5 -blue-green, which is weakly acidic to 4.5 - light yellow, which is strongly acidic represents states from mildly deficient to strongly deficient, respectively. Most children are dark blue, a pH of

7.5. Over half adults are green-yellow, a pH of 6.5 or lower, reflecting the calcium deficiency of aging and lifestyle habits. Terminal cancer patients are usually a bright yellow, a pH of 4.5. this is over 1000 times the acidity level of a normal healthy individual at pH 7.5, causing the body to self-digest. Also, acidic pH is exhibited by anxious and depressed adults, hyperactive children, and rebellious or delinquent adolescents. Psychologically, when a child sees that he is green, he will do almost anything to be blue like his buddies, especially if they watched him being tested. The same is true for adults, especially when the test has any yellow. This test is extremely believable, as it provides demonstrable proof of biophysical change. What you should know about the pH Test

The test, although generally reflective of the state of health of the patient, may not always be accurate. For example, while it is easier to test the pH of saliva than the pH of the blood, due to the ease of acquiring a sample, the saliva pH could be influenced by some recently consumed food, thereby producing a false positive test. This can be overcome by waiting for two hours after placing anything in the mouth before taking the test.

The patient should also draw fresh saliva into the mouth and swallow it, several times before taking the test. Also, because of a temporary aberration in the body, such as an adjustment for an overconsumption of some food high in some contributing component such as phosphates or alcohol, the pH could be temporarily affected.

Thus, an acidic test should be retested two hours later. If still acid, a good nutritional practice would be to adopt a good mineral and vitamin therapy, change of lifestyle, more oxygen intake (mild exercise) and exposure to full spectrum lighting. This should also be accompanied by change of diet to more fresh organic fruit, vegetables, fresh raw whole cream milk, eggs, and moderation in red meat (rich in phosphates) and alcohol. Avoid soft drinks, and in general, choose food known to be nutritious, remembering that anything, no matter how good it is supposed to be, is bad in excess.

Above all take it easy and try and relax, as you are embarking on a new course of action that can set your biological clock back a few notches, allowing you to lead a healthier, active and fulfilling life.

Remember that the total environment, emotional and physical, in which we function, effect the biochemical

Appendix E
Amino Acids

This information is a breakdown of the amino acid and enzymes profile found in the sea mineral formula described in chapter 4.

"The importance of balancing the amino acids to obtain the best possible protein from foods, cannot be over stressed." John D. Kirschmann, Author - "Nutrition Almanac"

Amino acids are more plentiful than any other substance in the body, next to water. They are one of the most important elements for the maintenance of good health and vitality and are of primary importance in the growth and development of all body components. All the tissues, bones and nerves are made up mostly of Amino Acids. They are the major source of building material for muscles, blood, skin, hair, nails and internal organs, including the heart and the brain.

Essential Amino Acids

Isoleucine

Isoleucine is an amino acid formed during hydrolysis of fibrin and other proteins. It is essential in the diet. Needed for hemoglobin formation and also stabilizes and regulates blood sugar levels.

Leucine

Promotes the healing of bones, skin and muscles and is recommended for those recovering from surgery. This amino acid aids in increasing growth hormone production. It is present in the body tissues and is essential for normal growth and metabolism.

Lysine

Improves concentration and mental alertness. Utilizes fatty acids required in energy production. It also helps to control herpes simplex outbreaks. It is essential for growth and repair of tissues.

Methionine

Is a powerful antioxidant. It is a good source of sulfur, which deactivates dangerous free radicals in the body. Also, helps in the breakdown of fats and helps reduce edema.

Phenylalanine

Enhances sexual interest, improves memory and alertness. Very useful in alleviating symptoms of premenstrual syndrome (PMS) and is a very strong anti-depressant.

Threonine

Helps to maintain the proper protein balance in the body. It enhances the immune system by aiding the production of antibodies. Also helps the liver function more efficiently.

Tryptophan

Combats stress, depression, insomnia and aids in weight control. Research reports it helps relieve migraine headaches and may reduce some of the harmful effects of nicotine. It is necessary for normal growth and development. Tryptophane is a precursor of serotonin, a neurotransmitter in the central nervous system.

Valine

Needed for muscle metabolism, tissue repair and the maintenance of proper nitrogen balance in the body. The muscles use it as a primary energy source. Derived from digestion of proteins.

Alanine

Aids in the metabolism of glucose, a simple carbohydrate that the body uses for energy.

Arginine

Metabolizes body fat and tones muscle, increases sperm count in males, aids in the healing of wounds and has been shown to retard the growth of tumors and cancer.

Aspartic Acid

Improves stamina and endurance, increases

resistance to fatigue, and helps protect the central nervous system. Low levels of this amino acid results in chronic fatigue syndrome.

Citrulline

Promotes energy, stimulates the immune system and detoxifies ammonia, which damages all living cells. This amino acid also helps keep the liver functioning properly.

Cysteine

Is the chief protein constituent of the fingernails, toenails, skin and hair. Aids in the production of collagen and promotes the proper elasticity and texture of the skin.

Cystine

Helps to detoxify the system, aids in protection from smoke, alcohol and heavy metals. It also helps protect the body against X-rays and nuclear radiation.

Glutamic Acid

Is the main neurotransmitter of the brain and spinal cord. Helps correct personality disorders and depression. It is also used in the treatment of epilepsy and Attention Deficit Disorder (ADD).

Glutamine

Used primarily as a brain fuel (improves intelligence). Alleviates fatigue and is also helpful in the treatment of arthritis, connective tissue diseases and fibromyalgia.

Glycine

Retards muscle degeneration, relieves gastric hyperactivity and has been successfully used in the treatment of manic (bipolar) depression and can also help diminish hyperactivity.

Histidine

Essential for the growth and repair of tissues and is vital to the production of both red and white blood cells. This amino acid helps protect the body from radiation damage, aids in removing heavy metals from the system and may help in the prevention of AIDS. Some authorities believe Histidine should be considered an essential amino acid.

Ornithine

Necessary for proper immune system and liver function. This amino acid also detoxifies ammonia and helps skin stay healthy. Accelerates tissue repair and wound healing.

Proline

Improves skin texture by aiding in the production of collagen and reducing wrinkles associated with aging. Also helps in the healing of cartilage, joints and tendons.

Serine

Aids in the production of immunoglobulins and antibodies that enables a healthy immune system. It is used as a moisturizing agent in many cosmetics and skin care preparations.

Taurine

Is the key component of bile, which is needed for the digestion of fats, the absorption of fat-soluble vitamins and the control of serum cholesterol levels.

Tyrosine

Regulates moods and combats depression. It suppresses the appetite and helps reduce body fat. Very successful in combatting Chronic Fatigue Syndrome and Narcolepsy.

Enzymes

"The length of life is in direct proportion to the rate of exhaustion of the enzyme potential of an organism. The increased use of food enzymes promotes a decreased rate of exhaustion of the enzyme potential."

Dr. Edward Howell Author - "Enzyme Nutrition"

Enzymes - The Spark of Life

Enzymes are involved in every life process in the body. They are an essential link in stamina, energy level, and ability to utilize vitamins, minerals and other nutrients, as well as contributing to the immune system's ability to protect our health.

Plant enzymes are the most important factor in maintaining radiant health and vitality. A secret to staying young and healthy, enzymes work on a digestive level and metabolically (throughout the body). Lack of enzymes contributes to disease and chronic degenerative conditions. With assimilation impaired, absorption of putrefying matter can occur throughout the body. Thus, an unhealthy body lacks resistance to germs, which proliferate in this environment.

Working on all pH levels (2.5-9), these enzymes affect the length and quality of life by breaking down old cellular mucous and toxins, then expelling it from the organism. Inflammation can be reduced, while immune system activity is increased. Enzymes are essential for digesting food, stimulating the brain, providing cellular energy and repairing all tissues, organs and cells. Each enzyme has a specific function in the body that no other enzyme can fulfill.

The enzymes in sea vegetation enable the various areas of the cells to perform at their maximum cellular metabolic rate and aid in the natural unlocking and unbinding of minerals, making them available and more efficiently useful at a cellular level. Some enzymes assist the cells in various organs and tissues to create and manufacture the hormones necessary for body function, such as corticosteroids from the adrenal cortex, growth hormones from the pituitary gland and androgens from the testes.

The enzymes found in sea vegetation also aid in the binding withdrawal and removal of numerous toxic chemicals and residues, which have accumulated in our bodies. Without enzymes the body would never utilize the food we ingest.

Amylase	**Lipase**
Breaks down Carbohydrates	Breaks down Fat
Cellulase	Protease
Breaks down Cellulose Fiber	Breaks down Protein

Glossary

Alimentary - of or relating to the function of nutrition.

Alimentary canal - the passage in the body through which food travels, comprising the mouth, pharynx, esophagus, stomach and intestines, and which serves digestion, absorption of food and the elimination of solid waste products.

Amino Acid - any of a large group of organic acids containing a carboxyl group, COOH, and an amino group, NH2. Each molecule contains an amino (&NH2) and an acid (&COOH) group. Any group of the 25 amino acids that link together into chains to form proteins that are necessary for all life; in general, they are water-soluble, crystalline, amphoteric (reacting chemically either as an acid or a base) electrolytes; ten of these (essential amino acids) cannot be synthesized by the human body but must be consumed. The molecules from which proteins are constructed.

Amphoteric - having both acid and base properties.

Anion - an ion carrying a negative charge; the opposite of cation. An anion is attracted by, and travels to, the anode (positive pole of an electrical source). Examples are acid radicals and corresponding radicals of their salts.

Anticoagulant - a substance that delays or prevents the clotting of blood.

Antioxidant - a substance that slows down the oxidation of hydrocarbons, oils, fats etc., and thus helps to check deterioration; (a substance which inhibits unwanted oxidation by being oxidized itself before other vital substances are affected).

Atom - the smallest part of an element. An atom consists of a nucleus (which contains protons and neutrons) and surrounding electrons. The nucleus is positively charged, and this determines the atomic number of an element.

Carbohydrates - are a basic source of energy. They are stored in the body as glycogen in virtually all tissues, but principally in the liver and muscles. Carbohydrates can be mobilized from those sites, making these stores an important source of reserve energy.

Carboxyl - the characteristic group COOH of organic acids, including fatty acids and amino acids.

Catalase - an enzyme found in blood and other tissues that decomposes hydrogen peroxide into water and free oxygen.

Cation - an ion with a positive electric charge (a positively charged ion); opposite of anion. In electrolysis, cations move toward the cathode - it is attracted by the cathode (negative pole).

Cell membrane - the membrane that surrounds the cytoplasm of a cell and serves as both a container and a sentry gate to effect admission, rejection, retention, or expulsion of various substances.

Chelate - a chemical compound in which the central atom (usually a metal ion) is attached to neighboring atoms by at least two coordinate bonds in such a way as to form a closed chain. A trace mineral bound to an amino-acid molecule. From the Greek word for "claw."

Collagen -a strong, fibrous insoluble protein found in connective tissue, including the dermis, tendons, ligaments, deep fascia, bone, and cartilage. Collagen is a network of fibrous protein which structurally supports the cells of the body; it is the most abundant protein in mammals, constituting a quarter of the total protein. Collagen is the protein typical of dental tissues (except enamel). Collagen fibers also form the periodontal ligament, which attaches the teeth to their bony sockets.

Colloid - coined by T. Graham (1805 - 1860), a Scot chemist. A solid, liquid, or gaseous, glue-like substance, such as a protein or starch, whose particles (molecules or aggregates of molecules), when dispersed as much as possible in a solvent, remain uniformly distributed and do not form a true solution. A substance made up of very small, insoluble, non-diffusible particles (as single large molecules or masses of smaller molecules) that remain in suspension in a surrounding solid, liquid, or gaseous medium of different matter. A state of matter consisting of such a substance dispersed in a surrounding medium. All living matter contains colloidal material, and a colloid has only a negligible effect on the freezing point, boiling point, or vapor pressure of the surrounding medium. The iodine-containing, glutinous protein stored in the thyroid. A small crystalloid grain of protein found in some cells, seeds etc.

Crystalloid - a substance capable of crystallization, which in solution, readily passes through vegetable and animal membranes. The opposite of colloid.

Cyclic - of, or relating to, a major group of organic compounds, structured in closed chains and having a ring-shaped structure.

Cytoplasm - the viscous substance that surrounds the cell nucleus.

DNA (deoxyribonucleic acid) - the substance mainly within the chromosomes of a cell that contains the genetic information. The information for making all the RNA (ribonucleic acid) and all the proteins of the body is stored in the DNA (it contains the genetic code and transmits the hereditary pattern).

Electrolyte - any substance which, in solution or in a liquid form, is capable of conducting an electric current by the movement of its dissociated positive and negative ions to electrodes. A substance that, in solution, conducts an electric current and is decomposed by its passage. Acids, bases, and salts are common electrolytes. An ionized salt in blood, tissue fluids, and cells. Acids, bases, and salts are common electrolytes. An ionized salt in blood, tissue fluids, and cells. These salts include sodium, potassium, and chlorine.

Electron - an extremely minute particle with a negative electrical charge that revolves about the central core or nucleus of an atom. Its mass is about 1/1840 g. The number of electrons circulating around a nucleus is equal to the number of positive charges on the nucleus.

Element - Traditionally, any of four substances - earth, air, fire, and water. In chemistry, a substance that cannot be separated into substances different from itself by ordinary chemical processes. Elements exist in free and combined states. Elements found in the human body include oxygen, aluminum, carbon, hydrogen, nitrogen, calcium, phosphorus, potassium, sulfur, sodium, chlorine, magnesium, iron, fluorine, iodine, copper, manganese, and zinc.

Endocrine -any gland that produces secretions that are distributed in the body by way of the bloodstream (ductless glands).

Enzymes - large protein molecules that act as organic catalysts which regulate virtually every chemical reaction in the organism.

Free radical - a molecule with an unpaired electron. The stability varies widely depending on the structure, but the more unstable free radicals there are, the more they participate in extended chain reactions which can damage the cell.

Free-radical deactivator - any substance that prevents harmful reactions of free radicals in the body by reacting with the radicals themselves and forming relatively harmless compounds.

Genetic Engineering - the synthesis, alteration, and/or replacement of genetic material by artificial means.

Histamine - an amine, $C_5H_9N_3$, produced by the carboxylation of histidine and found in all organic matter, functioning in the regulation of blood pressure and gastric secretion, etcetera, and released by certain cells in allergic reactions.

Homeostasis - the tendency of the body to maintain normal, internal chemical and functional equilibrium by means of regulating mechanisms initiated primarily by the hypothalamus (a primitive portion of the brain located between the two large hemispheres and influencing many basic body functions.)

Hydrocarbon -a compound made up primarily of hydrogen and carbon.

Hydrolysis - literally, to split with water, the breaking of a chemical bond with the resultant addition of a molecule of water.

Hypertension - raised blood pressure. Having greater than normal tension or tone.

Hypoglycemia - a disorder characterized by low tolerance to normal or elevated blood-sugar levels and resulting in sudden, steep drops of blood sugar.

Hypothalamus - a primitive portion of the brain located between the two large hemispheres and influencing many basic functions, such as temperature, blood pressure, hunger, thirst, and heart rate, by secreting releasing factors, which affect the pituitary gland.

Hypoxia - Deficiency in the amount of oxygen reaching body tissues.

Iatrogenic - caused by medical treatment; said especially of symptoms, ailments, or disorders induced by drugs or surgery.

Intracellular - of or occurring within individual cells.

Integrity - having an undiminished or unimpaired state. Ethical purity. The quality or state of being complete, unbroken condition, wholeness, entirety.

Ion - an atom or group of atoms that has lost one or more electrons and has a positive charge, or has gained one or more electrons and has a negative charge.

In aqueous solutions, ions are called electrolytes because they permit the solution to conduct electricity. Positive ions such as sodium, potassium, magnesium, and calcium are called cations; negative ions such as chloride, bicarbonate, and sulfate are called anions. In body fluids, ions are available for reactions (e.g. calcium ions from food may be combined with carbonate ions to form calcium carbonate, part of bone matrix).

Krebs cycle -(Sir Hans Krebs - 1900-1981, co-winner of a Nobel Prize in 1953) . A cyclic series of biochemical reactions that represents the final common pathway in all aerobic organisms for the oxidation of amino acids, fats, and carbohydrates, and also converts the citric acid, etc. from food into carbon dioxide and ATP (a key energy-carrying molecule in biological systems) energy. It is the main pathway of terminal oxidation in the process of which not only carbohydrates but proteins and fats are utilized.

Ligand - an atom, group, ion, radical, or molecule which forms a coordination complex with a central atom or ion. An organic molecule attached to a central metal ion by multiple bonds.

Metabolic - of, involving, characterized by, or resulting from metabolism.

Metabolism -the chemical and physical processes continuously going on in living organisms and cells, consisting of anabolism and catabolism. All energy and material transformations that occur within living cells, the sum of all physical and chemical changes that take place within an organism. It includes material changes (i.e., changes undergone by substances during all periods of life, such as growth, maturity, and senescence) and energy changes (i.e., all transformations of chemical energy of foodstuffs to mechanical energy or heat). Metabolism involves two fundamental processes: anabolism and catabolism. Anabolism is the conversion of food molecules into living cells and tissue; catabolism is the breakdown of complex chemicals into simpler ones, often producing waste products to be excreted, catabolism also includes cell respiration for the release of heat energy and formation of ATP; it is formed when energy is released from food molecules during cell respiration..

Microgram (mcg) -a measure of weight equivalent to a millionth of a gram; 1kg (kilogram) = 2.2lbs or 1,000g (grams); 1g = 1,000mg (milligrams); 1mg = 1,000 mcg.

Molecule - the smallest particle of an element or compound that can exist in the free state and still retain the characteristic of the element or compound: the molecules of elements consist of one atom or two or more similar atoms; those of compounds consist of two or more different atoms.

Any electrically neutral aggregate of atoms held together strongly enough to be considered as a unit. The individual atoms in the molecule may be of the same type or different. Combinations of dissimilar atoms form chemical compounds. The positive and negative charges balance exactly. Excess or deficiency of either positive or negative charge by the loss or acquisition of electrons results in the formation of an ion. A molecule is designated by the number of atoms it contains, as monatomic (one atom); diatomic (two); triatomic (three); tetratomic (four); pentatomic (five); or hexatomic (six).

Neutralize - to destroy the distinctive or active properties of an alkali - neutralize an acid. To make electrically neutral, to make inert.

Neurotransmitter - a biochemical substance that transmits or inhibits nerve impulses at a synapse (the minute space between a nerve cell and another nerve cell, a muscle cell, etcetera, through which nerve impulses are transmitted from one to the other).

Ozone - a highly reactive form of oxygen consisting of three oxygen atoms (O3) as compared to breathable oxygen, which has two atoms (O2), and produced by a high-voltage electrical discharge in air.

Parenteral - brought into the body as by subcutaneous (just beneath the skin) or intravenous (IV) injection.

pH - [p(otential of) h(ydrogen).] a measure of the hydrogen ion concentration of a solution. In chemistry, the degree of acidity or alkalinity of a substance are expressed in pH values. A solution that is neither acid nor alkaline is neutral and has a pH of 7. Increasing acidity is expressed as a number less than 7, an increasing alkalinity as a number greater than 7. Maximum acidity is pH 0 and maximum alkalinity is pH 14. Because the pH scale is logarithmic, there is a 10fold difference between each unit. For example, pH 5 is 10 times as acid as pH 6 and pH 4 is 100 times as acid as pH 6. The pH of a solution may be determined electrically by a pH meter or color-metrically by the use of indicators.

RNA (ribonucleic acid) - a nucleic acid that is an essential component of all cells, composed of a long, usually single stranded chain. RNA is a substance similar to DNA, which derives genetic information from DNA in order to construct proteins.

Sulfur amino acid - any amino acid that contains sulfur.

Synergistic - pertaining to the interaction of two or more agencies (often drugs) which, together, produce a greater total effect than the sum of their individual effects.

References and Recommended Reading
Books

Aebi E, Wyss SR, "Acatalasemia" in The Metabolic Basis of Inherited Disease (5th Edition) Stanbury JB, et al, eds. (McGraw-Hill, New York, 1983), pp. 1421-2

Affany A, et al, Fund Clin Pharmacol 1(1987): 451-7; Das N, Ratty A, "Effects of Flavonoids on induced Non-Enzymatic Lipid Peroxidation" in Plant Flavonoids In Biology and Medicine, Vol. 1(Alan R. Liss, Inc., New York, 1986), pp. 243-7

American Academy of Dental Science. (1876) *A History of Dental and Oral Science in America* (Dexter, J.E., ed) S.S. White Publ., Philadelphia.

American Academy of Dental Science. (1876) *A History of Dental and Oral Science in America* (Dexter, J.E., ed) S.S. White Publ., Philadelphia

American Dental Association Divisions of Communication and Scientific Affairs (1990) When your patients ask about mercury in amalgam. *J. Am. Dent. Assn.* 120, 395 - 398

American Dental Association Divisions of Communication and Scientific Affairs (1990) When your patients ask about mercury in amalgam. *J. Am.*

Dent. Assn. 120, 395-398

American Medical Association Council on Food and Nutrition, NUTRIENTS IN PROCESSED FOODS, ACTION, Mass: Publishing Sciences Group, 1974.

Ames BN, et al, Proc Natl Acad Sci USA 78(1981): 6858-62

Ames BN, Shigenaga MK, "DNA Damage by Endogenous Oxidants and Mitogenesis As Causes of Aging and Cancer" in *Molecular Biology of Free Radical Scavenging Systems,* Scandalios JG, ed. (Cold Spring Harbor Laboratory Press, Plainview, 1992), pp. 1-21

Ames BN, Shigentaga MK, "DNA Damage by Endogenous Oxidants and Mitogenesis As Causes of Aging and Cancer" in Molecular Biology of Free Radical Scavenging Systems, Scandalios JG, ed. (Cold Spring Harbor Laboratory Press, Plainview, 1992),pp.1-21

An authoritative standard reference work "the pharmacological basis of therapeutics," Louis Goodman, Alfred Gillman NY, McMillan, 1970 states " caffeine induces chromosomal breakage in the fruit fly, higher plants and a variety of microorganisms ...It has similar affects in man."

An authoritative standard reference work "the pharmacological basis of therapeutics," Louis Goodman, Alfred Gillman NY, McMillan, 1970 states " caffeine induces chromosomal breakage in the fruit fly, higher plants and a variety of microorganisms ... It has similar affects in man."

Aposhian, H.V., Bruce, D.C., Alter, W., Dart, R.C., Hurlbut, K.M., and Aposhian, M.M. (1992) Urinary mercury after administration of DMPS: correlation with dental amalgam score *FASEB J.* 6, 2472 - 2476

Aposhian, H.V., Bruce, D.C., Alter, W., Dart, R.C., Hurlbut, K.M., and Aposhian, M.M. (1992) Urinary mercury after administration of DMPS: correlation with dental amalgam score. *FASEB J.* 6, 2472-2476

Aronsson, A. M., Lind, B., Nylander, M., and Nordberg, M. (1989) Dental amalgam and mercury. *Biol. Metals* 2, 25 - 30

Aronsson, A.M., Lind, B., Nylander, M., and Nordberg, M. (1989) Dental amalgam and mercury. *Biol. Metals* 2, 25- 30

Ashmead DeWayne, H, Ph.D., Graff Darrell, J, Ph.D., Ashmead Harvey, H, Ph.D. "Intestinal Absorption of Metal Ions and Chelates (Charles Thomas Publisher. Springfield, Illinois 1985)

Backer, W. E. (1973) Geochimica et Cosmochimica Acta, 37, 269-281

Barnes, S., M.D., et al, THE ROLE OF SOY PRODUCTS IN REDUCING RISKS OF CANCER, National Journal of Cancer, Vol, 83, No. 8, P. 541, April 17, 1991.

Baumann J, et al, Prostanglandins 20(1980): 627-39; Hsieh R, et al, Lipids 23(1988): 322-6

Beisel WR, Am J Clin Nutr 35 (supplement) (1982): 417-8

Beladi I, et al, Ann NY Acad Sci 284(1977): 238-64

Bendich A, et al, Adv Fee Radic Biol Med 2(1986): 419-44

Berry, T. G., Nicholson, J. and Troendle, K. (1994) Almost two centuries with amalgams; Where are we today? *J. Am. Dent. Assn.* 125, 392 - 399

Berry. T.G., Nicholson, J. and Troendle, K. (1994) Almost two centuries with amalgam: Where are we today? *J. Am. Dent. Assn.* 125, 393-399

Biology of Aging: Gene Stability and Gene Expression, Sohal RS, et al, eds. (Raven Press, new York, 1985), pp. 307-40

Blazso G, Gabor M, Acta Physiol Acad Sci (Hungary)

56(1980): 235-40

Block, K.I., M.D., THE EFFECT OF DIET ON QUALITY AND QUANTITY OF LIFE IN CANCER PATIENTS, Symposium, adjuvant Nutrition for Cancer Patients, Nov. 6, 1992, Tulsa, Ok.

Block, K.I., M.D., THE EFFECT OF DIET ON QUALITY AND QUANTITY OF LIFE IN CANCER PATIENTS, Symposium, Adjuvant Nutrition for Cancer Patients, Nov. 6, 1992, Tulsa, Ok.

Bloomfield, V.A., Crothers, D.M., and Tinoco, I., Jr. (1974) *Physical Chemistry Nucleic Acids,* pp, 420 - 429, Harper & Row Publ., New York

Bloomfield, V.A., Crothers, D.M., and Tinoco, I., Jr. (1974) *Physical Chemistry Nucleic Acids*, pp. 420-429, Harper & Row Publ., New York Magos, L., Halbach, S., and Clarkson, T.W. (1978) Role of catalase in the oxidation of mercury vapor. *Biochem. Pharmacol.* 27, 1373-1377

Borunov EV, et al, *Biull Eksp Biol Med* 107(1989): 467-9 (Russian, with English Abstract)

Boyd, N.D., Benediktsson, H., Vimy, M.J., Hooper, D.E., and Lorscheider, F.L. (1991) Mercury from dental "silver" tooth fillings impairs sheep kidney function. *Am. J. Physiol.* 261, R1010 - R1014

Boyd, N.D., Benediktsson, H., Vimy, M.J., Hooper, D.E., and Lorscheider,

Bremmer, M.D.K. (1954) *The Story of Dentistry, #rd. Ed.,* Dental Items of Interest Publ. Co., Brooklyn.

Bremner, M.D.K. (1954) *The Story of Dentistry, 3rd Ed.,* Dental Items of Interest Publ. Co., Brooklyn

Brown MS, Goldstein JL, *Annu Rev Biochem* 52(1983): 223-661; Kita T, et al, *J Clin Invest* 77(1986): 1460-5; Steinberg D, *Arterioscl* 3(1983): 283-301; Goldstein JL, et al, *J Cell Biol* 82(1979): 597-613; Fogelman AM, et al, *Proc Nat'l Acad Sci* USA 77(1980):2214-8

Buffle, J. (1988). Complexation Reactions in Aquatic Systems: An Analytical Approach. Chichester: Horwood.

Burger RM, et al, *Life Sci* 28 (1981): 715-27; Lin PS, et al, *Cancer* 46(1980): 2360-4

Burkitt, D., Towell, H.C., WESTERN DISEASES; THEIR EMERGENCE AND PREVENTION, Cambridge, Mass: Harvard University Press, 1981.

Burrell CJ, Blake DR, *Br Heart J* 61(1989): 4-8; Davies SW, "Free Radicals and Myocardial Disease-Studies in Patients" in *Free Radicals, Diseased States and Anti-Radical Interventions,* Rice-Evans C, ed. (Richelieu Press, London, 1989), pp. 97-115

California Fertilizer Association. (1985). Western Fertilizer Handbook. Danville, Il: Interstate.

Carney JM, et al, *Proc Nat'l Acad Sci* USA 88(19910: 3633-6

Chaboussou, F. (1980). Les Plantes Malades des Pesticides -Bases Nouvelles D'une Prevention Contre Maladies et Parasites. (Plants made sick by pesticides - New basis for the prevention of diseases and pests). Paris.

Chemical Nature Of The Water Barrier", A. Molottsy, J. Of Invest. Derm. 1968, No. 50, PP 19-20.

Chlorinated drinking water is directly responsible for more than 4,200 cases of bladder cancer and 6,500 cases of rectal cancer every year. These figures are based on a study published in the American Journal of Public Health (AJPH) just a couple of years ago. Chlorine reacts with other substances in water to form chloroform, carbon tetrachloride and

Chlorinated drinking water is directly responsible for more than 4,200 cases of bladder cancer and 6,500 cases of rectal cancer every year. These figures are based on a study published in the American Journal of Public Health (AJPH) just a couple of years ago. Chlorine reacts with other substances in water to form chloroform, carbon tetrachloride and other cancer-causing compounds. The study was conducted by the Medical College of Milwaukee.

Chlorinated Organics During Water Disinfection", Scully Environ, SCI. Technol., Vol 22, No 5, 1988, 537-542

Christman, R.F., & Gjessing, E. T. (1983). *Aquatic and Terrestrial Humic Materials*. The Butterworth Grove, Kent, England: Ann Arbor Science.

Ckarlson, T.W., Hursh, J.B., Sager, P.R., and Syversen, T.L.M. (1988) Mercury. In *Biological Monitoring of Toxic Metals* (Clarkson, T.W., Friberg, L., Nordberg, G.F., and Sager, P.R., eds) pp. 199-246. Plenum, New York

Clarkson, T.W., Friberg, L., Hursh, J.B., and Nylander, M. (1988) The prediction of intake of mercury vapor from amalgams. In *Biological Monitoring of Toxic Metals* (Clarkson, T.W., Friberg, L., Nordberg, G.F., and Sager, P.R., eds) pp. 247 - 260. Plenum, New York

Clarkson, T.W., Friberg, L., Hursh, J.B., and Nylander, M. (1988) The prediction of intake of mercury vapor from amalgams. In *Biological Monitoring of Toxic Metals* (Clarkson, T.W., Friberg, L., Nordberg, G.F.,

Clarkson, T.W., Hursh, J.B., Sager, P.R., and Syversen,

T.L.M. (1988) Mercury. In *Biological Monitoring of Toxic Metals* (Clarkson, T.W., Friber, L., Nordberg, G.F., and Sager, P.R., eds) pp. 199 - 246 Plenum, New York

Cotran RS, et al, eds., Robbins Pathologic Basis of Disease (W.B. Saunders Co., Philadelphia, 1989), pp. 25-6, 686-8

Crapo JD, McCord JM, Am J Physiol 231(1976): 1196-1203

Cross CE, et al, *Ann Intern Med* 107(1987): 526-45

Cutler RG, "Longevity is Determined by Specific genes: Testing the Hypothesis" in *Testing the Theories of Aging,* Adelman R, Roth G, eds. (CRC Press, Boca Raton, 1982), pp. 25-114; Cutler RG, "The Dysdifferentiative Hypothesis of Mammalian Aging and Longevity" in *The Aging Brain: Cellular and Molecular Mechanisms of Aging in the Nervous System,* Aging vol. 20, Giacobini E, et al, eds. (Raven Press, New York, 1982), pp. 1-19; Cutler RG, "Dysdifferentiation and Aging' in *Molecular*

Cutler RG, Am J Clin Nutr 53(1991): 373S-9S

D.L. (1994) The molecular basis of microtubule stability in neurons. *Neurotoxicology,* 15, 109 - 122

Danscher, G., Horsted-Bindslev, P., and Rungby, J.

(1990) Traces of mercury in organs from primates with alamgam fillings. *Exp. Mol. Pathos.* 52, 291-299

Dariel, M.P., Lashmore, D.S., and Ratzker, M. (1994) New technology for mercury free metallic dental restorative alloys. *Powder Metallurgy,* 37, 88

Davies KJ, et al, Biochem Biophys Res Comm 107(1982): 1198-205

de Duve C, A Guided Tour of Living Cell, Vol. 1, (Scientific American Library, New York, 1984), pp.180-7

Dean Burk, 1941. On the specificity of glycolysis in malignant liver tumors as compared with homologous adult or growing liver tissues. In Symposium of Respiratory Enzymes, University of Wisconsin Press. pp. 235-245. 1942. Dean Burk, Science 123, 314, 1956. Woods, M.W., Stanford, K.K., Burk, D., Earle, W.R. J. National Cancer Institute 23, 1079-1088, 1959. Dean Burk. Burk, D., Woods, M. and Hunter, J. On the significance of Glucolysis for Cancer Growth, with Special Reference to Morris Rat Hepatomas. Journ. National Cancer Institute 38, 839-863, 1967.

del Maestro RF, et al, "Free Radicals and Micorvascular Permeability" in *Pathology of Oxygen,* Autor AP, ed. (Academic Press, New York, 1982), pp. 157-73;

Fligiel SEG, et al, *Fed Proc* 43(1984): 954 (Abstract)

Demopoulos HB, et al, "Oxygen free Radicals in central Nervous system Ischemia and Trauma" in *Pathology of Oxygen*, Autor AP, ed. (Academic Press, New York, 1982), pp. 127-55

DeWall RA, et al, *Am Heart F* 82(1971): 362-70; Lefer AM, et al, *Circ Shock* 8(1981): 273-82, McCord, *Can*); Fantone, *Current*

Diet, Nutrition, and Cancer National academy Press, Washington, D.C., 1982)

Diplock At, *Am J Clin Nutr* 53(1991): 189S-93S; Niki E, et al, *Am J Clin Nutr* 53(1991): 201S-5S; Di Mascio P, et al, *Am J Clin Nutr* 53(1991): 194s-200S; Luc G, Fruchart J-C, *Am J Clin Nutr*, 53(1991): 206S-9S

Diplock AT, Am J Clin Nutr 53(1991): 189S-93S; Niki E, et al Am J Clin Nutr 53(1991): 201S-5S; Di Mascio P, t al Am J Clin Nutr 53(1991): 194S200S

Diplock, *Am F* (see note 6); Niki, *Am F* (see note 6); Di Mascio, *Am F* (see note 6): Luc, *Am F* (see note 6); Weisburger JH, *Am F Clin Nutr* 53(19910: 226S-37S

Dr. Allen E. Banik and Renée Taylor. Hunza Land (Whitehorn Publishing, Long Beach, CA. 1960)

Drasch, G., Schupp, Il, Hofl, H., Reinke, R., and Roider, G. (1994) Mercury burden of human fetal and infant tissues. *Eur. J. Pediat.* 153, 607-610

Druet, P., Bernard, A., Hirsch, F., Weening, J.J., Gengoux, P., Mahieu, PP., and Berkeland, S. (1982) Innumologically medicated glomerulonephritis induced by heavy metals. *Arch. Toxicol.* 50, 187 - 194

Duhr, E., Pendergrass, C., Kasarskis, E., Slevin, J., and Haley, B. (1991) Hg^{2+} induces GTP-tubulin interactions in rat brain similar to those observed in Alzheimer's disease. *FASEB J.* 5, A456

Duhr, E.F., Pendergrass, J.C., Slevin, J.T. and Haley, B.E. (1993) HgEDTA complex inhibits GTP interactions with the E-site of brain B-tubulin. *Toxicol. Appl. Pharmacol.* 122, 273 - 280

Duhr, E.F.,Pendegrass, J.C., Slevin, J.T. and Haley, B.E. (1993) HgEDTA complex inhibits GTP interactions with the E-site of brain B-tubulin. *Toxicol. Appl. Pharmacol.* 122, 273-280

Emanuel NM, "Free Radicals during Appearance and growth of Tumors" in *Free Radicals and Cancer,* Floyd RA, ed. (Marcel Dekker, Inc., New York, 1982), pp. 245-319; Shulyakovskaya TA, et al, *Dokl Akad Nauk,* USSR 210(1973): 221-3

Emerit I, Michelson AM, *Proc Nat'l Acad Sci USA*

78(1981): 2537-40

Ernest L. Wynder, Sven Hultberg, Folke Jacobsson, and Irwin J. Bross, Environmental Factors in Cancer, Cancer, Vol. 10, 470, 2057.

Escheverria, D., Heyer, N., Martin M.D., Naleway, C.A., Woods, J.S., and Bittner, A.C. (1995) Behavioral effects of low level exposure to Hg^0 among dentists. *Neurotoxicol. Teratol.* 17, 161 - 168

Escheverria, D., Heyer, N., Martin, M.D., Naleway, C.A., Woods, J.S., and Bittner, A.C. (1995) Behavioral effects of low level exposure to Hg^0 among dentists. *Neurotoxicol. Teratol.* 17, 161-168

F.L. (1990) Whole-body imaging of the distribution of mercury released from dental fillings into monkey tissues. *FASEB J.* 4, 3256 - 3260

F.L. (1991) Mercury from dental "silver" tooth fillings impairs sheep kidney function. *Am. J. Physiol.* 261, R1010-R1014

Fackelmann KA, Sci News 138(1990): 333

Fahn S, *Am F Clin Nutr* 53(19910: 380S-2S

Falconer, N.M., Vaillant, A., Reuhl, K.R., Laferriere, N., and Brown, D.L. (1994) The molecular basis of microtubule stability in neurons. *Neurotoxicology*, 15, 109-122

Fantone JC, Ward PA, *Current Concepts: Oxygen-Derived Radicals and Their Metabolites: Relationship to Tissue Injury* (The Upjohn Company, Kalamazoo, 1985), p. 36

Farrington JA, et al, *Biochim Biophys Acta* 314(1973): 372-81; Pyatak PS, et al, *Res Commun Chem Pathol Pharmacol* 29(1980): 113-27; Fisher HK, et al, *Ann Intern Med* 75(1971): 731-6; Ishida, *Biochem* (see note 40); Sugiura, *F Biol* (see note 40); Ferrans, *Adv* (see note 41); von Hoff, *Am* (see note 41); Lefrak, *Cancer* (see note 41)

Ferrans VJ, *Adv Exp Med Biol* 161(1983): 519-32; Von Hoff DD, et al, *Am F Med* 62(1977): 200-8; Lefrak EA, et al, *Cancer*

Forman HJ, Fisher AB, "Antioxidant Defenses" in Oxygen and Living Processes, Gilbert DL, ed. (Springer-Verlag, New York, 1981), pp. 23572; Lubin b, Machlin LJ, eds. "Vitamin E: Biochemical, Hematological and Clinical Aspects" New York Academy of Sciences, Annals, Vol. 393 (1982)

Freeman BA, et al, J Biol Chem 258(1983): 12534-42

Fridovich I, "Oxygen Radicals, Hydrogen Peroxide, and Oxygen Toxicity" in Free Radicals in Biology, Vol. 1, Pryor WA, ed. (Academic Press, New York, 1976), pp. 239-77

Fridovich I, "Superoxide Dismutase in Biology and Medicine" in Pathology of Oxygen, Autor AP, ed. (Academic Press, New York, 1982), pp.1-19

G. Cameron, J. Exper. Med. 97, 525, 1953.

Gay, D.D. and Cox, R.D. (1981) The effects of dental amalgams on mercury levels in expired air. *J. Dent. Res.* 60, 1668-1671

Gilbert, M. P., and Summers, A. O. (1988) The distribution and divergence of DNA sequences related to the Tn21 and Tn501 meroperons. *Plasmid* 20, 127 - 136

Gilbert, M.P., and summers, A.O. (1988) The distribution and divergence of DNA sequences related to the Tn21 and Tn501 mer operons. *Plasmid* 20, 127- 136

Gillian Martlew, N.D., *Electrolytes the Spark of Life* (Nature's Publishing, Florida, 1998)

Goering, P.L., Galloway, D.W., Clarkson, T.W., Lorscheider, F.L., Berlin, M., and Rowland, A.S. (1992) Toxicity assessment of mercury vapor from dental amalgams. *Fundam. Appl. Toxicol.* 19, 319 - 329

Gonzalez-Ramirez, D., Maiorino, R.M., Zuniga-Charles, M., Xu, Z., Hurlbut, K.M., Junco-Munoz, P., Aposhian, M.M., Dart, R.C., Gama, J.H.D.,

Escheverria, D., Woods, J.S., and Aposhian, H.V. (1995)

Gonzalez-Ramirez, D., Maiorino, R.M., Zuniga-Charles, M., Xu, Z., Hurlbut, K.M., Junco-Munoz, P., Aposhian, M.M., Dart, R.C., Gama, J.H.D., Escheverria, D., Woods, J.S., and Aposhian, H.V. (1995) Sodium 2,3-dimercaptopropate-1-sulfonate (DMPS) challenge test for mercury in humans: II - Urinary mercury, porphyrins and neurobehavioral changes of dental workers in Monterrey, Mexico. *J. Pharmacol. Exp. Ther.* 272, 264274

Goto Y, "Lipid Peroxides as a Cause of Vascular Diseases" in *Lipid Peroxides in Biology and Medicine,* Yagi K, ed. (Academic Press, New York, 1982), pp. 295-303

Graf, E., M.D., THE ROLE OF SOY PRODUCTS IN REDUCING RISKS OF 0CANCER, National Journal of Cancer, Vol. 83, No. 8, p. 544, April 17, 1991.

Graham S, et al, Am J Epidem 113(1981): 675-7

Greenland, D. J.. (1965). Soils and Fertilizers. 35(5), 415-532.

Greenwald RA, Moy WW, *Arthritis Rheum* 23(1980): 455-63

Gregory Em, Fridovich I, J Bacteriol 114(1973): 543-8

Grogaard B, et al, *Am J Physiol* 242(1982): G448-54

Gross, M.J., and Harrison, J.A. (1989) Some electrochemical features of the *in vivo* corrosion of dental amalgams. *J. Appl. Electrochem.* 19, 301-302

Gross, M.J., and Harrison, J.A. (1989) Some electrochemical features of the *in vivo* corrosion of dental amalgams. *J. Appl. Electrochem.* 19, 301-310

Guarnieri C, et al, *J Mol Cell Cardiol* 12(1980): 797-808

Guyton AC, *Textbook of Medical Physiology, Eight Edition* (W.B. Saunders Co., Philadelphia, 1991), pp. 819-30

Hahn, L.J., Kloiber, R., Vimy, M.J. Takahashi, Y., and Lorscheider, F.L. (1989) Dental "silver" tooth fillings: A source of mercury exposure revealed by whole-body image scan and tissue analysis. *FASEB J.* 3, 2641-2646

Hahn, L.J., Kloiber, R., Leininger, R.W., Vimy, M.J., and Lorscheider, F.L. (1990) Whole-body imaging of the distribution of mercury released from dental fillings into monkey tissues. *FASEB J.* 4, 3256-3260

Hahn, L.J., Kloiber, R., Vimy, M.J., Takahashi, Y., and Lorscheider, F.L. (1989) Dental "silver" tooth fillings: A source of mercury exposure revealed by whole-body image scan and tissue analysis. *FASEB*

J. 3, 2641-2646

Halliwell B, "Free Radicals, Oxygen Toxicity, and Aging" in *Age Pigments,* Sohal RS, ed. (Elsevier--North Holland Biomedical Press, Amsterdam, 1981), pp. 1-662; Halliwell B, *Bull Europ Physiopath Resp* 17 (Supplement)(1981): 21-9

Halliwell B, Bull Europ Physiopath Res 17(1981) (Supplement): 21-9; Dormandy TL, "Ceruloplasmin and serum Antioxidant Activity" in Oxygen free Radicals and Tissue damage, Gilbert DL, ed. (Excerpta Medica, New York, 1979), pp. 166-8

Harman D, "The Free-Radical Theory of Aging" in *Free Radicals in Biology, Vol. 5,* Pryor WA, ed. (Academic Press, New York 1982), pp. 2255-75

Heart and Stroke Facts (American Heart Association, 1991)

Hendler SS, The Complete Guide to Anti-Aging Nutrients (Simon and Schuster, New York, 1984), p.88; Harris RWC, Brit J Cancer 53(1986): 653-9; Shekelle RB, et al, Lancet 2(1981): 1185-90

Henry A. Schroeder, M.D., The Trace Elements and Man. (Devine-Adair Company, Old Greenwich, Connecticut. 1973)

Hirsch, F., Kuhn, J., Ventura, M., Vial, M-C., Fournie,

G., and Druet, P. (1986) Autoimmunity induced by HgCl2 in Brown-Norway rats. I. Production of monoclonal antibodies. *J. Immunol.* 136, 3272-3276

Hooper C,*J NIH Res* 1(1989): 101-6; Stringer M, et al, *Br Med J* 298(1989): 281-4

Hultman, P., Johansson, U., Turley, S.J., Lindh, U., Enestrom, S., and Pollard, K.M. (1994) Adverse immunological effects and autoimmunity induced by dental amalgam and alloy in mice. *FASEB J.* 8, 1183 -1190

Hultman, P., Johansson, U., Turley, S.J., Lindh, U., Enestrom, S., and Pollard, K.M. (1994) Adverse immunological effects and autoimmunity induced by dental amalgam and alloy in mice. *FASEB J.* 8, 1183-119

Human Biochemistry, 5th ed. Kliener and Orten, page 389 Organic Chemistry. 3rd ed. Morrison and Bpvd, page 584 "Vitamin E a re-examination." Horwitt M.K. Ph.D., Am. J. Clin. Nutr. 29:569-578 "Absorption and Retention of vitamin E Com. in Ad. Humans." Horwitt

Ingalls, T.H. (1983) Epidemiology, etiology and prevention of multiple sclerosis. *Am. J. Forensic Med. Path.* 4, 55- 61

Ishida R, Takahashi T, *Biochem Biophys Res Commun* 66(1975): 14328; Sugiura Y, Suzuki T, *F Biol Chem* 257(1982): 10544-6

Iwu M, "Biflavanones of Garcinia: Pharmacological and Biological Activities" in Plant Flavonoids In Biology and Medicine, vol. 1 (Alan R. Liss, Inc., New York, 1986), pp. 485-8

J Food Sci 51(1986): 1009-13; Shamberger R, Nutrition and Cancer (Plenum Press, New York, 1984); Bracke M, et al, "Flavonoids Inhibit Malignant Tumor Invasion In Vitro" in Plant Flavonoids In Biology and Medicine, vol. 2(Alan R. Liss, Inc., New York, 1988), pp. 219-33

Jackson, William R. (1993). Humic, Fulvic and Microbial Balance: Organic Soil Conditioning. Evergreen, Colorado: Jackson Research Center.

Jacobs, M. R., Ph.D., FOOD COMPONENTS WITH THERAPEUTIC POTENTIAL, Symposium Adjuvant Nutrition for Cancer Patients, Nov. 6, 1992, Tulsa, Ok.

John A. Mann, Secrets of Life Extension (And/Or Press, Inc, Berkeley, CA and Harbour Publishing, San Francisco. 1980)

Khatoon, S., Campbell, S.R., Haley, B.E., and Slevin,

J.T. (1989) Aberrant guanosine triphosphate-B-tubulin interaction in Alzheimer's disease. *Ann. Neurol.* 26, 210 - 215

Khatoon, S., Campbell, S.R., Haley, B.E., and Slevin, J.T. (1989) Aberrant guanosine triphosphate-B-tubulin interaction in Alzheimer's disease. *Ann. Neurol.* 26, 210-215

Kita T, "Lipoprotein Metabolism in the WHHL Rabbit; An Animal Model for Familial Hypercholesterolemia" in *Atherosclerosis VII*, Fidge NH, Nestel PJ, eds. (Elsevier, Amsterdam, 1986), pp. 227-30; Yokode M, et al, in *Advances in Prostaglandin, Thromboxane and Leukotriene Research*, Samuelsson B, et al, eds. (Medical and Scientific Publishers, New York, 1987)

Klaassen, C.D. (1990) Heavy Metals and heavy-metal antagonists. In *the Pharmacological Basis of Therapeutics, 8th Ed.* (Gilman, A.G., Rall, T.W., Nies, A.S., and Taylor, P., eds) pp. 1598-1602, Pergamon Press, New York

Klaassen, C.D. (1990) Heavy metals and heavy-metal antagonists. In *The Pharmacological Basis of Therapeutics, 8th Ed.* (Gilman, A.G., Rall, T.W., Nies, A.S., and Taylor, P., eds) pp. 1598 -1602, Pergamon Press, New York

Kononova, M. M. (1966). Soil Organic Matter. Elmsford, NY: Pergamon.

Krinsky NI, "Biological Roles of Singlet Oxygen" in Singlet Oxygen, Wasserman HH, Murray RW, eds. (Academic Press, New York, 1979), pp. 597-641; Singh A, et al, Bull Europ Physiopath Resp 17(1981) (Supplement): 31-41; Singh A, Can J Physiol Pharmacol 60(1982): 2330-45

Kronhausen e, et al, *formula for Life* (William Morrow and Co., Inc., New York, 1989), p.76

Kronhausen E, et al, Formula for Life (William Morrow and Company, New York 1989), p.77

Larsson A, et al, eds., Functions of Glutathione: Biochemical, Physiological, Toxicological, and clinical Aspects (Raven Press, New York, 1983)

Leibovitz BE, Nutrition Update 6 (1992): 1-15

Leibovitz BE, Nutrition Update 6(1992): 181-6

Levine SA, Kidd PM, Antioxidant Adaptation: Its Role in Free Radical Pathology (Biocurrents Division, Allergy research group, San Leandro, 1986),p.49

Levine SA, Kidd PM, *Antioxidant Adaptation: Its Role in Free Radical Pathology* (Biocurrents Division, Allergy Research Group, San Leandro, 1986),p. xi

Lorscheider, F.L., Vimy, M.J., Pendergrass, J.C., and Haley, B.E., (1994) Toxicity of ionic mercury and elemental mercury vapor on brain neuronal protein metabolism. 12th International Neurotoxicology Conference, Hot Springs, AR October 31, 1994. *Neurotoxicology.* 15, 955

Lorscheider, F.L., and Vimy, M.J. (1993) Evaluation of the safety issue of mercury release from dental fillings. *FASEB J.* 7, 1432-1433

Lorscheider, F.L., and Vimy, M.J. (1993) Evaluation of the safety issue of mercury release form dental filling. *FASEB J.* 7, 1432 - 1433.

Lorscheider, F.L., Vimy, M.J., Pendergrass, J.C., and Haley, B.E. (1994) Toxicity of ionic mercury and elemental mercury vapor on brain neuronal protein metabolism. 12th International Neurotoxicology Conference, Hot Springs, AR, October 31, 1994. *Neurotoxicology,* 15, 955

Luc, *Am J Clin Nutr* (see note 6); Riemersma RA, et al, *Lancet* 337(1991): 1-5; Jialal I, et al, *Atherosclerosis* 82(1900): 185-91

Lvstad RA, Int J Biochem 13(19810: 221-4; Denko CW, Agents Actions 9 (1979), pp.166-8

M.K. Ph.D., Fed. of Amer. Soc. Exp. Bio. 84

Machin J, Bendich A, FASEB J 1(1987):441

Magos, L., Halbach, S., and Clarkson, T.W. (1978) Role of catalase in the oxidation of mercury vapor. *Biochem. Pharmacol.* 27, 1373 - 1377

Malcolm, R. D., & Vaughan, D. (1979). Comparative effects of soil organic matter fractions on phosphatase activities in wheat roots. Plant and Soil, 51, 117-126. Also: Mato, M. C., Gonzales-Alonso, L. M.,& Mendez, J. (1972). Inhibition of enzymatic indoleacetic acid oxidation by fulvic acids. Soil Biology and Biochemistry, 4, 475-478.

Maridonneau I, et al, *J Biol Chem* 258(1983): 3107-13

Masi, J.V. (1995) Corrosion of amalgams in restorative materials: the problem and the promise. In *Status Quo and Perspectives of Amalgam and other Dental Materials* (Frieberg, L., Schrauzer, G.N., eds) ThiemeVerlag, Stuttgart.

Masi, J.V. (1995) Corrosion of amalgams in restorative materials: the problem and the promise. In *Status Quo and Perspectives of Amalgam and other Dental Materials* (Friberg, L., Schrauzer, G.N., eds) Thieme Verlag, Stuttgart. In press

Mead JF, "Free Radical Mechanism of Lipid Damage and Consequences for Cellular Membranes" in *Free*

Radicals in Biology, Vol. 1, Pryor WA, ed. (Academic Press, New York, 1976), pp. 51-68

Meerson FZ, et al, *Biull Eksp Biol Med* 92(1981): 281-3 (Russian, with English abstract); Davies SW, et al, *Lancet* 335(1990): 741-3

Meister, A., and Anderson, M.E. (1983) Glutathione. *Ann. Rev. Biochem.* 52, 711 - 760

Menkes MS, et al, N Eng J Med 315(1986): 1250-89

mercury in organs from primates with amalgam fillings *Exp. Mol. Pathol.* 52, 291 - 299

Messina, M., Ph.D., Barnes, S., M.D. et al, THE ROLE OF SOY PRODUCTS IN REDUCING RISKS OF CANCER, National Journal of Cancer, Vol., 83, No. 8, P. 541-544, April 17, 1991.

Molin, M., Bergman, B., Marklund, S.L., Schutz, A., and Skerfving, S. (1990) Mercury, selenium and glutathione peroxidase before and after amalgam removal in man. *Acta Odontol. Scand.* 48, 189 - 202

Molin, M., Bergman, B., Marklund, S.L., Schutz, A., and Skerfving, S. (1990) Mercury, selenium and glutathione peroxidase before and after amalgam removal in man. *Acta Odontol. Scand.* 48, 189-202

Morel DW, et al, *Arterioscl* 4(1984): 357-64; Steinbrecher UP, et al, *Proc Nat'l Acad Sci* USA 77(1980): 2214-8

Niwa Y, Hanssen M, *Protection for Life: How to boost Your Body's Defences Against Free Radicals and the Ageing Effects of Pollution and Modern Lifestyles* (Thorsons Publishers, Ltd., Wellingborough, 1989),

Niwa Y, Tsutsui D, Saishinigaku (Japan) 38(1983): 1450-8

Novi AM, Science 212(1981): 541-2

Nylander, M., Friberg, L., and Lind, B. (1987) Mercury concentration in the human brain and kidneys in relation to exposure from dental amalgam fillings. *Swed. Dent. J.* 11, 179 - 187

Nylander, M., Friberg, L., and Lind, B. (1987) Mercury concentrations in the human brain and kidneys in relation to exposure from dental amalgam fillings. *Swed. Dent. J.* 11, 179-187

O. Warburg, New Methods of Cell Physiology, Georg Thieme, Stuttgart, and Interscience Publishers, New York, 1962.

Ochsner A, et al, JAMA 144(1950): 831-4; Ochsner A, N Eng J Med 271(1964): 211(letter)

O'Halloran, T.V. (1993) Transition metals in control of gene expression. *Science* 261, 715-725

Organic Compounds (VOCS) In Drinking Water," Halina Brown, American Journal of Public Health,

Vol 74, 5/84

Otto Warburg, A.W. Geissler, and S. Lorenz: Über die letzte Ursache und die entfernten Ursachen des Krebses, 17. Mosbacher Kolloquium, April 1966. Verlag Springer, Heidelberg 1966.

Otto Warburg, Heavy Metals as prosthetic groups of enzymes, Clarendon Press, Oxford, 1949.

Oxygen free Radicals and Tissue Damage (Ciba Foundation Symposium

P. (1986) Autoimmunity induced by HgCl2 in Brown-Norway rats. I. Production of nomoclonal antibodies. *J. Immunol.* 136, 3272 - 3276

Palkiewicz, P., Zwiers, H., and Lorscheider, F.L. (1994) ADP-ribosylation of brain neuronal proteins is altered by *in vitro* and *invivo* exposure to inorganic mercury. *J. Neurochem.* 62, 2049-2052

Patterson, J. E., Weissberg, B., and Denninson, P.J. (1985) Mercury in human breath from dental amalgam. *Bull. Environ. Contam. Toxicol.* 34, 459-468

Pauling L, How to live Longer and feel Better (W.H. Freeman & Company, New York, 1986), pp. 173-9

Pecora P, Shriftman MS, *A Study of Insulin, Fatty Acids and Other Metabolites in Psychiatric and Normal Control Populations* (Monroe Medical Research Laboratory,

Monroe, 1983)

Ponomareva, V. V., & Ragim-Zade, A. I. (1969). Comparative study of fulvic and humic acids as agents of silicate mineral decomposition. Society Soil Science, 1, 157-165. (Trans. From Pochvovedenie. (1969), 3, 26-36).

Prakash, A. (1971). Fertility of the Sea, 2, 351-368.

Rashid, M.A. (1985). Geochemistry of Marine Humic Substances. New York: Springer-Verlag.

Reinhardt, J. W. (1988) Risk assessment of mercury exposure from dental amalgams. *J. Pub. Hlth. Dent.* 48, 172 - 177.

Reinhardt, J.W. (1988) Risk assessment of mercury exposure from dental amalgams. *J. Pub. Hlth. Dent.* 48, 172-177

Richard G.cutler, Biochemist, National Institute on Aging, personal communication (June 1992)

Ring, M.E. (1985) *Dentistry: An Illustrated History.* H.N. Abrams Inc. Publ., New York.

Robert R. Barefoot and Carl J. Reich, M.D. The Calcium Factor (Triad Marketing, 2002)

Roehm JN, et al, Arch Environ Health 24(1972): 237-42; Mustafa MG, Nutr Rep Int 11(1975): 475-81; Fletcher

BL, Tappel AL, Environ Res 6(1973): 165-75

Roney PL, Holian A, *Toxicol Appl Pharmacol* 100(1989): 132-44

Rowland, A.S., Baird, D.D., Weinberg, C.R., Shore, D.L. Shy, C.M., and Wilcox, A.J. (1994) The effect of occupational exposure to mercury vapour on the fertility of female dental assistants. *Occup. Environ. Med.* 51, 28-34

Salk, P. L., & Parker, L. W. (1986). A New Agricultural Biotechnology: Potential Applications in Arid and Semi-Arid Zones. American Association for the Advancement of Science and the Government of LaRioja, Argentina.

Salonen JT, et al, Brit Med J 290(1985): 417-20

Sato Y, et al, *Biochem Med* 21(1979): 104-7

Saylor B, Arch Otolaryngol 50(1949): 813-20; Schoenkerman B, Justice R, Ann Allergy 10(1952): 138-41

Seligman ML, et al, *Lipids* 12(1977): 945-50

Senesi, N. (1990) Analytica Chimica Acta, 232, 51-75. Amsterdam, The Netherlands: Elsevier.

Senesi, N. (1990). Molecular and quantitative aspects of the chemistry of fulvic acid and its interactions with metal ions and organic chemicals: Bari Italy. Analytica Chimica Acta, 232, 51-75. Amsterdam, The Netherlands: Elsevier.

Shamberger R J, et al, Arch Environ Health 31(1976): 231-5; Schrauzer GN, et al, Bioinorg Chem 7(1977): 23-31; Schrauzer GN, et al, Bioinorg Chem 8(1978): 303-18; Mondragon MC, Jaffe WG, Arch Latinoamer Nutr 26(1976): 341-52

Shamberger RJ, et al, *Arch Environ Health* 31(1976): 231-5; Schrauzer GN, et al, *Bioinorg Chem* 7(19977): 23-31

Shute WE, Taub HJ, Vitamin E for Ailing and Healthy Hearts (Pyramid House, New York, 1969)

Simonson, R. W. (1959). Outline of a generalized theory of soil genesis. Soil Science Society America Proceedings, 23, 152-156

Skare, I., and Engqvist, A. (1994) Human exposure to mercury and silver released from dental amalgam restorations. *Arch. Environ. Hlth.* 49, 384 - 394

Skare, I., and Engqvist, A. (1994) Human exposure to mercury and silver released from dental amalgam restorations. *Arch. Environ. Hlth.* 49, 384- 394

Smith GS, Walford RL, *Nature* 270(1977): 727-9; Williams RM, et al, "Genetics of Survival in Mice:

Localization of Dominant Effects to subregions of the Major Histocompatibility Complex" in *Immunological Aspects of Aging,* Segre D, smith L, eds. (Dekker Publishing Company, New York, 19810: 247-66

Sodium2,3-dimercaptopropane-1-sulfonate (DMPS) challenge test for mercury in humans: II - Urinary mercury, porphyrins and neurobehavioral changes of dental workers in Monterrey, Mexico. *J. Pharmacol. Exp. Ther.* 272, 264 - 274

Southorn P, Powis G, *Mayo Clin Proc* 63(1988): 390-408

Spittle CR, Lancet 2(1973): 199-201 (letter); Sarji KE, et al, Thrombosis Research 15(1979): 639-50; Bordia AK, Atherosclerosis 35 (1980): 181-7; Cardova C, et al, Atherosclerosis 41(1982):15-9

Stringer, *Br Med*(see note 17); Cotran RS, et al, eds., *Robbins Pathologic Basis of Disease* (W.B. Saunders Co., Philadelphia, 1989)

Summers, A. O., Wireman, J., Vimy, M.J., Lorscheider, F.L., Marshall, B., Levy, S.B., Bennett, S., and Billard, L. (1993) Mercury released from dental "silver" fillings provokes an increase in mercury-and antibiotic-resistant bacteria in oral and intestinal floras of primates. *Antimicrob. Agents & Chemother.* 37, 825 - 834

Svare, C.W., Peterson, L. C., Reinhardt, J.W., Boyer, D.B., Frank, C.W., Gay, D.D. and Cox, R.D. (1981) The effects of dental amalgams on mercury levels in expired air. *J. Dent. Res.* 60, 1668 - 1671

Tanaka K, Sugahara K, Plant Cell Physiol 21(1980): 601-11; Rabinowitch HD, et al, Arch Biochem Biophys 225 (1983):640-8

Tappel Al, "Measurement of and Protection From in vivo Lipid Peroxidation: in Free Radical in Biology, vol. IV, Pryor WA, ed. (Academic Press, New York, 1980),pp. 1-47; Dillard CJ, et al, J Appl Physiol 45(1978): 927-32

Taubald RD, et al, *Lipids* 10(1975): 383-90

The Environmental Protection Agency (EPA) learned that chlorinated water decreases the "good" cholesterol (HDL) and increases the bad cholesterol (LDL). Therefore you increase the risk of heart disease as well as the risk of cancer at the same time.

The Environmental Protection Agency (EPA) learned that chlorinated water decreases the "good" cholesterol (HDL) and increases the bad cholesterol (LDL). Therefore you increase the risk of heart disease as well as the risk of cancer at the same time.

The Journal of Nutrition (November 1949) reported that Dr. Clive M. McCay and assistant Lois Will, (Cornell University) stated that cola drinks would erode i.4 mlgs of calcium per gram of tooth in three hours. A study with mice fed on soda like solution of phosphororic acid and sucrose (which is in colas) : after six months on diet the rats' teeth eroded away to the gum.

Thompson, C.M., Markesbery, W.R., Ehmann, W.D., Mao, Y. - X. and Vance, D.E. (1988) Regional brain trace-element studies in Alzheimer's disease. *Neurotoxicology* 9, 1 - 7

Till GO, et al, *J Clin Invest* 69(1982): 1126-35; Johnson A, et al, *Am J Pathol* 114(1984: 410-7; Ward PA, et al, *J Clin Invest* 72(1983): 789801; Perkowski SZ, et al, *Circ Res* 53(1983): 574-83; Till GO, et al *J Trauma* 23(1983): 269-77

U.S. Department of Agriculture, Food Technology, 1981, p. 9, 35

U.S. News & World Report, July 29, 1991, PP. 48-55.

Villar A, et al, J Pharmacy Pharmacol 36(1984): 820-3

Vimy, M.J. and Lorscheider, F.L. (1985) Intra-oral air mercury released from dental amalgam. *J. Dent. Res.* 64, 1069-1071

Vimy, M.J., and Lorscheider, F.L. (1985) Serial measurements of intraoral air mercury: Estimation of daily dose from dental amalgam. *J. Dent. Res.* 64, 1072-1075

Vimy, M.J., and Lorscheider, F.L. (1990) Dental amalgam mercury daily dose estimated from intra-oral vapor measurements: A predictor of mercury accumulation in human tissues. *J. Trace Elem. Exp. Med.* 3, 111-123

Vimy, M.J., and Lorscheider, F.L., (1990) Dental amalgam mercury daily dose estimated from intra-oral vapor measurements: A predictor of mercury accumulation in human tissues. *J. Trace Elem. Exp. Med.* 3, 111 - 123

Vimy, M.J., Takahashi, Y., and Lorscheider, F.L. (1990) Maternal-fetal distribution of mercury (203 Hg) released from dental amalgam fillings. *Am. J. Physiol.* 258, R939 - R945

Vimy, M.J., Takahashi, Y., and Lorscheider, F.L. (1990) Maternal-fetal distribution of mercury (203-Hg) released from dental amalgam fillings. *Am. J. Physiol.* 258, R939-R945

Walford RL, *Maximum Life Span* (Avon, New York, 1983), p. 168

Wattenberg L, Leong J, Can Res 30(1970): 1922-55; Marwan A, Nagel C,

Wattenberg, can (see note 84); Kuttan R, et al, Experientia 37(1981): 221-3

Weiss SJ, LoBuglio AF, *Lab Invest* 47(1982): 5-18: Fantone JC, Ward PA, *Am F Pathol* 107(1982): 395-418

Weitzman SA, et al, *Science* 227(1985): 1231-3: Southorn, *Mayo*

Wenstrup, D., Ehmann, W.D., and Markesbery, W.R. (1990) Trace Element imbalances in isolated subcellular fractions of Alzheimer's disease brains. *Brain Res.* 533, 125-131

Wenstrupp, D., Ehmann, W.D., and Markesbery, W.R. (1990) Trace element imbalances in isolated subcellular fractions of Alzheimer's disease brains. *Brain Res.* 533, 125 - 131

Werbach, M., M.D., COMPARING THE RISK TO BENEFIT RATIO OF DRUGS AND NUTRIENTS, Symposium, Adjuvant Nutrition for Cancer Patients, Nov. 6, 1992, Tulsa, Ok.

Whalley CV, et al, Biochem Pharmacol 39(1990):1743-50

Wilkins, M.D. (Ed.). (1984). Advanced Plant Physiology. Marshfield, MA: Pitman.

Williams, Dr. Roger J. (1977). The Wonderful World Within You. Bio-Communications Press. Wichita, Kansas.

Willstaetter, Wieland and Euler, Lectures on enzymes at the centenary of the Gesellschaft Deutscher Naturforscher. Berichte der Deutschen Chemischen Gesellschaft, 55, 3583, 1922. The three lectures of the three chemists show that in the year 1922 the action of all enzymes was still a mystery,. No active group of any enzyme was known.

World Health Organization (1991) *Environmental Health Criteria 118, Inorganic Mercury* (Friberg, L., ed) WHO, Geneva

X-RAYS PROVED DANGEROUS -*from* **Public Scrutiny**, *April 1982, page 6* WASHINGTON--Dr. John Gofman, Gofman makes his case in a new, 908-page book, "Radiation and Human Health,"

Yagi K, "Assay for Serum Lipid Peroxide Level and its Clinical Significance" in *Lipid Peroxides in Biology and Medicine,* Yagi K, ed (Academic Press, New York, 1983), pp. 223-42

Yasukawa K, et al, "Effect of Flavonoids on Tumor Promoter's Activity: in Plant Flavonoids In Biology and Medicine, Vol. 2 (Alan R. Liss, Inc., New York,

1988), pp. 247-50

Zalups, R.K. (1991) Autometallographic localization of inorganic mercury in the kidneys of rats: Effect of unilateral nephrectomy and compensatory renal growth. *Exp. Mol. Pathol.* 54, 10-21

Zalups, R.K., (1991) Autometallographic localization of inorganic mercury in the kidneys of rats : Effect of unilateral nephrectomy and compensatory renal growth. *Exp. Mol. Pathol.* 54, 10 - 21

Zalups, R.K., and Barfuss, D.W. (1990) Accumulation of inorganic mercury along the renal proximal tubule of the rabbit. *Toxicol. Appl. Pharmacol.* 106, 245-253

Articles

"Cancer Incidence And Trihalomethane Concentrations In A Public Drinking Water System", George L. Carlo, American Journal of Public Health, Vol 74, No. 5, 1984, pp. 479-484.

"Cancer Incidence And Trihalomethane Concentrations In A Public Drinking Water System", George L. Carlo, American Journal of Public Health, Vol 74, No. 5, 1984, pp. 479-484.

"Coronaries, Cholesterol, Chlorine", Joseph M. Price,

Jove Book, Alta Enterprises, 1969.

"Did You Know That --- A Long Hot Shower", Bottom Line Personal, Aug. 15, 1987

"Human Exposure To Volatile Organic Compounds In Household Tap Water, The Inhalation Pathway", T.E. McKone Environ, SCI, Technology, Vol 21, No. 12, 1987, PP. 1194-1201.

"Is Your Water Safe To Drink?", Raymond Gabler, Consumer Reports Book, 1987.

"Is Your Water Safe?", Carpenter, Hedges, Crabbe, Reilly and Bounds,

"Mademoiselle", prior to August 15, 1987.

"Non-Ingestion Exposure To Chemicals In Potable Water", Julian Andelman Working Paper 84-03, University of Pittsburgh, 1984.

"Organic Chemical Contaminants In Drinking Water, And Cancer", AM J. Epidemiology, Vol 110, 1979, P. 420

"Proteins In Natural Waters And Their Relation To The Formation Of Chlorinated Organics During Water Disinfection", Scully Environ, SCI. Technol., Vol 22, No 5, 1988, 537-542

"Regional Variation In Percutaneous Penetration In Man, Pesticides", H.J. Malback, Arch. Environ. Health, Vol. 23, Sept. 1971, P. 209.

"Showers Pose a Risk To Health", Ian Anderson, New Scientist, 9/18/86.

"Studies Of Diffusion Of Water Through Dead Human Skin, The Effect Of Different Environmental States And Of Chemical Alterations Of The Epidermis", G.S. Berenson and G.E. Burch, AM.J. Of Tropical Medicine, 1951, No.**Suggested Additional Reading Material**

Electrolytes the Spark of Life - Gillian Martlew, N.D., Nature's Publishing, Florida, 1998.

Tissue Cleansing Through Bowel Management, by Dr. Bernard Jensen

The Importance of Squatting, by William Welles, D.C.

The Culture of the Abdomen, 1924, author unknown

The Prevention of Diseases Peculiar to Civilization, Sir W. Arbuthnot Lane

Inflammation and Cancer, The Flavonoids: Advances in Research, 3rd edition by B. Harborne, Chapman and Hall, 1993.

Death by Diet, Robert R. Barefoot, Triad Marketing

These books briefly review several of the most basic aspects of molecular structure and activities in the cell- -information available in any basic textbook on the subject. For lay readers interested in further detail, I recommend books from the *Scientific American* series: Atkins PW, *Atoms, Electrons, and Change* (Scientific American Library, New York, 1991): Atkins PW, *Molecules* (Scientific American Library, New York, 1987); de Duve C, *A guided Tour of the Living Cell, Volumes 1 & 2* (Scientific American Library, New York, 1984). For more substance, an excellent university textbook, well organized and clearly written, is: Alberts B, et al, *Molecular Biology of the Cell* (Garland Publishing, inc., New York, 1983).

Patrick Störtebecker - Stockholm, in springtime 1982.

The author thanks the Wallace Genetic Foundation, the International Academy of Oral Medicine and Toxicology, the University of Georgia Research Foundation, and the National Institutes of Health, whose support of research contained in a number of the citations herein made this review possible.

The PRICE-POTTENGER FOUNDATION maintains a list of doctors and dentists acquainted with this research.

For more information, Dr. Meinig's 211 page book is also

available. It is loaded with details, photographs and practical information (He even explains in detail how a tooth that's had a root canal needs to be removed,

"Studies Of Epidermal Water Barrier, Part 2. Investigation Of The

"Temporal Variations In Trihalomethane Content Of Drinking Water", V.L. Smith, Environ. SCI & Technol., Vol 14, No 2, 1987, pp 190-196.

"The Nader Report - Troubled Waters On Tap", Duff Conacher and Assc Center to Study of Responsive Law, January 1988.

"The Role Of Skin Absorption As A Route Of Exposure For Volatile Organic Compounds (VOCS) In Drinking Water," Halina Brown, American Journal of Public Health, Vol 74, 5/84

"THMS In Drinking Water", J.A. Cotruvo, Environ. SCI & Technol., Vol. 15, No. 3, 1981, PP. 268-274.

"Toxic Showers And Baths", Janet Raloff, Science News, Vol 130, Page

"Volatile Synthetic Organic Chemicals (VOCS)", K.V.Dyke Water Technol. Vol. 13, No. 4, Apr. 1990, P. 38.

"Water Can Undermine Your Health", N.W. Walker

D.S., Norwalk Press, 1974.

"Water", John F. Ashton and Ronald S. Laura, Nature & Health, 1988.

"Your Body's Many Cries for Water," F. Batmanghelidj, M.D. Global Health Solutions 1992

About The Author

Dr. Jacob Swilling holds a Ph.D. in Clinical Nutrition with more than twenty five years research experience in biochemistry with a specialization in chronic illness, cancer and degenerative disease. He is internationally known for his advanced work in the field of Biological Medicine which developed into a working model at the Genesis West Clinic located in Playas de Tijuana, Baja California Mexico which he and his wife operated for more than ten years. This Clinic was regarded as the most advanced of its kind in the testing, evaluation and treatment of cancer and other chronic disease. Genesis West used the most advanced technology available in innovative programs particularly his Predictive Medicine Evaluation revealing Early Warning Detection of imbalances in the biochemistry, pH balance, biological, bioenergetic, and immune systems which he describes as "trends towards illness and disease."

As a result of an invitation from a medical group in Malaysia, he successfully initiated several projects in that country as well as Singapore and Bangkok, Thailand. These included acting as a consultant to medical groups to establish Integrated Health Care

Centers, a Research and Development Program that has over 40 registered Medical Clinics. The success of his work was described in the Sunday Star Newspaper, the Medical Tribune as well as in other Malaysian and Chinese Newspapers and Magazines.

The success of these programs emphasizes that early correction will avoid a later crisis. His work has led to the development of Integrated Health Care combining the best of Allopathic and Natural Medicine which he continues to develop with Medical Doctors and Clinics. Programs integrate Detoxification, Non-Toxic Dentistry, Chelation, Oxygen and Ozone Therapy, Therapeutic Nutrition, including Intravenous Therapy, pH Balance, and Bio-Energetic Medicine. Currently his Cancer Self-Help Support Program is being used by an increasing number of practitioners and patients, being coordinated by a team of practitioners at his know Your Options Wellness Center in Costa Mesa, Southern California.

Several publications have published articles written by Dr. Swilling including Explore, Natural Health Magazine, National Health Federation Magazine and Alive in Canada. These include articles describing his research experience relating to cancer and degenerative disease. His research experience, demonstrating the connection between amalgam fillings and root canals as a causal factor in the development of Cancer and Multiple Sclerosis, was given special attention.

Dr. Swilling is known as a key-note speaker at Health Conventions in the United States, Canada, Mexico, South Africa, Israel, Thailand, and Malaysia. He is also a guest speaker on Radio and TV.

His workshops at Health Conventions included: "Oncology Support Program for Cancer Patients, Family and Friends, Anti-Aging, Regeneration and Life Extension, New Dimensions in Biological Medicine," and his popular weekend seminar "The Causes, Prevention and Treatment of Illness and Disease."

Dr. Swilling has completed four comprehensive books: Minerals: Key to Vibrant Health and Life Force,

Cancer Self-Help Support Program, Diabetes: A Self-Help Solution, and Beyond Bypass and Chelation for Heart and Cardiovascular Disease.

Dr. Swilling is also a faculty member of the Global College Of Nutritional Medicine offering approved degree courses.

*

Email: kyopublishing@gmail.com

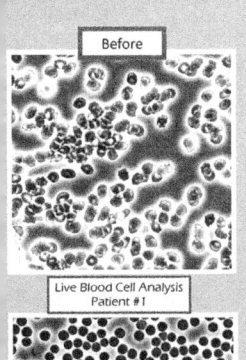

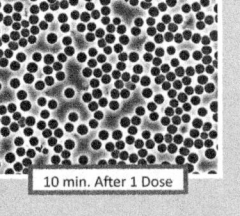

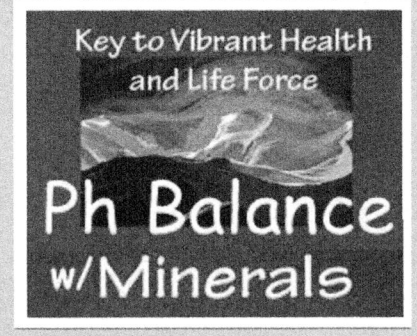

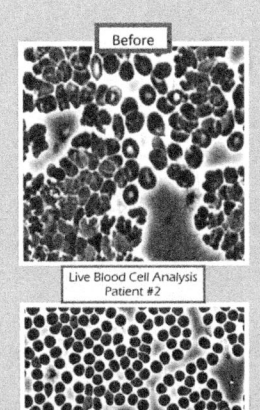

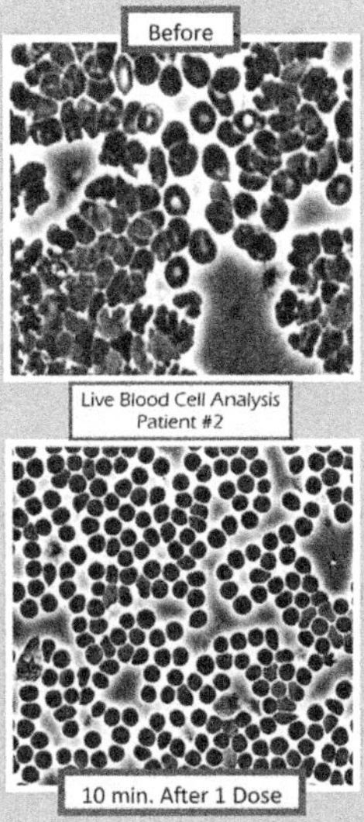

pH Balance With Minerals
A New ELECTROLYTE Breakthrough Minerals Product

Feel the impact aftero nly 2oz of minerals in a 16oz bottle 3 to 4 times daily!

Not all water delivers the same energy! The difference is the naturally occurring aquifer water found below the surface. Bottled at the site with 74 naturally occurring minerals, this product delivers maximum pH electrolyte power to restore pH balance at the cellular level.

Advanced Bio-Cell technology studies reveal that filtered city water alters surface tension and molecular structure so altering electrolyte delivery.

Feel The Difference!

For more information email kyopublishing@gmail.com

Printed in Great Britain
by Amazon